Your Esthetics Coach

An Esthetician's Guide to Success

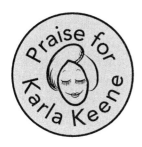

Praise for Karla Keene

Meet some of my Special Friends, Colleagues & Mentors that I have been Blessed to have worked with Throughout my Career...

"Meeting Karla in 2008 and working with her over the last seven years continues to be a wonderful and rewarding experience. Karla is a top-notch coach in the Esthetics industry. Her passion for skin care, ClarityRx® skin care products, and her talent to coach Estheticians with confidence, is a gift to the industry. Karla, thank you for all you do, for so many, many people."

John Marco
Founder, Hand & Stone Massage and Facial Spa Franchise

"Karla Keene IS the Esthetics business all wrapped up into one! She is THE pioneer and the leading educator in esthetics globally. She was an invaluable partner in my two successful medical spa ventures, both of which were successfully sold to private equity firms. Count on your own success when you choose to retain and work with Karla!"

John Buckingham
Entrepreneur and Marketing Professor, Pepperdine University

"Let me take the opportunity to say what a pleasure it has been to deal with you, Karla. You have been a rich resource. Your support, professionalism, and enthusiasm have been so motivating to me and my team."

Scott Creighton,
Vice President of New Ventures, Johnson & Johnson,
Consumer Products

"I have had the pleasure of working with Karla for over 20 years on various product development projects with some of the industry's largest personal care companies. Keene has an in-depth understanding of cosmetic ingredients and has developed creative, comprehensive and well-organized products and protocols for treating real skin problems. She is a master at the art of creating products from concept to consumer, and has an incredible way of providing sound education and training for best results."

Jerry Whittemore, PharmD
Cosmetic Chemist, Juniper Laboratories, Inc. Los Angeles, CA

"I have known Karla for over a decade. Her marketing expertise generated a multitude of sales for our company. By conducting highly successful seminars with our physicians, which offered training, marketing ideas and services, she was able to see us succeed. Some of Karla's success can be attributed to her strong organizational skills. Together with her talent for marketing and sales, she possesses the ability to increase the bottom line of any company she works with."

M.D. Former President exCel Cosmeceuticals
Bloomfield Hills, MI

"Karla is such a great educator! She makes everything so clear and easy to understand!"

Lucy Frost
Owner, Hand & Stone Massage and Facial Spa, Manalapan, NJ

"Karla Keene's Your Esthetics Coach is the go-to guide for all Skin Care Experts who want to be at the top of their field, providing all the tips and tools you need to follow your passion in the beauty industry. She has been my mentor for over a decade, inspiring me to take my career to levels I'd never dreamed of!"

Susie Augustin
Beauty Expert, Bestselling Author of Sexy, Fit & Fab at Any Age!

"Ms. Keene's mastery of the cosmeceuticals market, its products and their respective roles has contributed greatly to the foundation of knowledge upon which cosmeceuticals are built. I have no doubt that we owe a great part of the success of our sales representatives and company sales growth to Ms. Keene and her consistently accurate and always current portrayal of our changing market, its products and its ever increasing needs. Ms. Keene has played a huge role in the education and edification of our pharmaceutical and cosmeceutical sales staff and leaders. Her industry knowledge and honest and thorough representation of our customers' needs helps us stay focused on continuously meeting those needs."

C.G., Former Director of Marketing, Cosmetic Labs
Lake Forest, CA

"You are extremely knowledgeable and I was completely impressed by you! In my years in this business I have never had a trainer with your kind of experience. Thank you!"

M.N., Day Spa Owner,
Santa Cruz, CA

"I had the opportunity to meet Karla at a recent MedSpa owner's training class. The day I spent under her instruction was extremely informative. Her demeanor, expertise, and knowledge was second to none. The day ended too quickly! I look forward to learning more about the industry from Karla in the upcoming months. She will be an important part of my business!"

L.F., MedSpa Owner,
Broomfield, Colorado

"Thanks so much for an amazing training! The staff is still talking about how fabulous it was!"

C.L., MedSpa Owner
Boston, MA

"I wanted to THANK YOU again for the thorough training you provided to us at our MedSpa. You obviously made an impact on all of my team!"

L.S., MedSpa Owner
Houston, TX

"I have consulted and worked with Karla for several years. Her honesty, expertise, and vast knowledge of the aesthetic industry are one in a million. You know that you are getting the best of the best with Karla, to keep you and your company on the forefront of new products and technology, thus always staying ahead of the competition."

Janae Brand
Owner, Skinsultants Management Co., Los Angeles, CA

"Karla Keene, CEO and Founder of ClarityRx Clinical Skin Care, is the person who brought facials into the Hand & Stone Massage franchise in 2008. Through her amazing simple product line, continued education and support to all of our estheticians, Hand & Stone Massage Spa was transformed into Hand & Stone Massage and Facial Spa."

Maria A. Cermatori
Owner, Hand & Stone Massage and Facial Spa, Spring Lake, NJ

"Just wanted to thank you for a great seminar yesterday. I found the topics and the information valuable and walked away with a renewed feeling and more confidence. I hope to implement several key points into my interactions with clients."

N.B.
Licensed Esthetician

"Karla, It was such a pleasure meeting you this week. Your wealth of knowledge has made my first introduction into the esthetics industry so enjoyable, completely informative, as well as, just plain fun. I wish we had more time together!"

F.F., Retail Marketing Director
Long Island, NY

"I just wanted to thank you once again for all of the knowledge and the kindness that you showed. I am fortunate and blessed to have met people like you who can share their knowledge of the business and the trade with me!"

**K.M., Day Spa Owner,
Franklin, TN**

"Karla, thanks for everything. You are a very gracious professional and shared a lot with all of us. Everyone was impressed with your expertise!"

**N.W., MedSpa Owner,
Houston, TX**

"Karla has provided us with the best advice available in the industry. We are opening a med spa and it has been overwhelming to make the right decisions. Without Karla's help, we couldn't have done it. She has the inside scoop and the insight to give to her clients. We were able to save money and make decisions that will increase our bottom line. Thanks, Karla!"

**L.A., MedSpa Owner,
Pasadena, CA**

"It was certainly a pleasure meeting last week. Your presentation was extremely informative. We believe the right field support is critical in developing a successful business. We are comforted to know that we will have someone as knowledgeable and experienced as you supporting us with such an essential aspect of our business."

**B.S., MedSpa Owner,
West Palm Beach, FL**

"It was a pleasure meeting you. I was very impressed by you, your professionalism, and knowledge base. Thanks for a wonderfully educational day!"

J.G., M.D.
Plastic Surgeon, San Diego, CA

"We were thrilled with your training! One of my colleagues asked, "Who is this Karla person? She is all I have heard about!" Your ears must have been ringing! Thanks again!"

A.C., MedSpa Retail Marketing Director,
Nyack, NY

"All of us enjoyed having you here. The girls talked about it all day yesterday. They all learned so much from you and are very excited! Thank you so much, Karla! You've been wonderful and we all appreciate it so much."

S.R., MedSpa Owner,
Jacksonville, FL

"After working with Karla, my company began to grow in ways even I couldn't have imagined. Not only did I begin to visualize a whole new business sensibility, but also I began to tap into opportunities that have taken my company into new arenas of success. I credit my accomplishments in large part to Karla's superior knowledge and skill, but most of all to her overwhelming generosity and kindness. I know this is a relationship that will last longer than I am doing business…and the future is limitless with her and her team by my side."

C.M., Former President, Innovative Beauty,
Laguna Beach, CA

"I have had the pleasure of working with Karla for just a few short months and in that time I have found a real gem. Karla brings a wealth of experience and knowledge related to every aspect of the medical aesthetics market and has been a great asset to me. Her willingness to go above and beyond as she consults on every aspect of aesthetics makes her a real pleasure to work with and a valuable advisor to my business."

**P.C., MedSpa Owner,
La Costa, CA**

"Thank you for our esthetics training. You were awesome! Gosh, we were in awe of all of your knowledge."

**M.P., Marketing Director,
Colorado Springs, CO**

Your Esthetics Coach

An Esthetician's Guide to Success

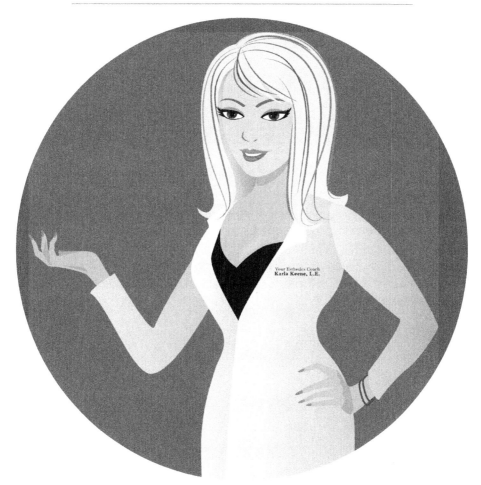

Karla Keene, L.E.

K² Publishing
Newport Beach, CA
www.YourEstheticsCoach.com

Limits of Liability and Disclaimer of Warranty.
The author and publisher shall not be liable for your misuse of this material. This book is strictly for informational and educational purposes.

Warning – Disclaimer.
The purpose of this book is to educate and entertain. The author and/or publisher do not guarantee that anyone following these techniques, suggestions, tips, ideas, or strategies will become successful. The author and/or publisher shall have neither liability nor responsibility to anyone with respect to anyone with respect to any loss or damage caused, or alleged to be caused, directly or indirectly by the information contained in this book.

ISBN 978-0-9967418-0-4 paperback

Library of Congress Cataloging-in-Publishing Data is available upon request.

Printed in the United States of America
First Printing, 2015

Edited by Get Branded Press www.GetBrandedPress.com
Cover & Interior Design by Kate Korniienko-Heidtman

Dedication

· · · · · · · · · · · · · · · · · · · ·

This book is dedicated to my son, Adam. Being his mom has taught me selflessness, compassion, drive, and love to a degree that I could have only imagined. He is what made me want to be successful. His patience and understanding of me as a person and as his mom, as I worked nonstop in an attempt to provide him with a full life, is indescribable. To my mom and dad for giving me the unconditional and solid foundation of love and support that allowed me to fly and not to fear. Thanks to my sister, Darcie, for being the best friend, confidante and business partner that I could ever ask for. To my extended family and friends for your encouragement and support along the way.

· · · · · · · · · · · · · · · · · · · ·

Acknowledgments

With over 33 years of experience as a licensed Esthetician and Educator, to finally write a book and to be able to download years of my experience and passion for the professional skin care industry, has always been a dream of mine. Susie Augustin, thank you for your friendship, inspiration, and encouragement in order for me to fulfill this dream. To my mentors that I have had the privilege of crossing divine paths with that have led me to this point in my career, you have all played an important role in my journey.

I would especially like to acknowledge my late, dear friend, Robert Diemer. You took me under your angel wings at such an early age of 19, and taught me absolutely everything that I needed to know to become a successful Esthetician, Educator and Business Owner throughout the extended time we worked together. Heaven took you way too soon. However, your infinite knowledge, endless empowerment, and deep passion for skin care lives on through me, and I am beyond grateful for the gift of having had you in my life. Although the industry knows you as the "Pioneer of Esthetics", you are forever my one and only true Esthetics Coach.

It is my hope to continue to educate and mentor Estheticians that share the same enthusiasm and passion as I do for our industry, just as I had the gift from my mentors. We all have a common goal...to continue to elevate our expertise and to perfect and preserve our profession. Here is to our continued journey and success together!

Cordially,
Karla Keene, L.E.
Your Esthetics Coach

TABLE OF CONTENTS

Foreword

Karla Keene's *Your Esthetics Coach* is the go-to guide for all Skin Care Experts who want to be at the top of their field, providing all the tips and tools you need to follow your passion in the beauty industry. She has been my mentor for over a decade, inspiring me to take my career to levels I'd never dreamed of!

It was so refreshing to meet another skin care expert who "did everything" – skin care education, sales, marketing, and product development. Karla did it all and made it all seem so effortless. She has a true passion for everything skin care! When Karla learned about my vast experience, she challenged me to continue to follow my passions, and take it up another notch. She suggested I look into marketing, branding and writing for skin care companies. I had the opportunity to work for her and travel the USA as a MedSpa Educator, and write and edit marketing and educational materials. A few years later in my forties, I went back to school to get my marketing degree, which led to employment at a beauty manufacturing company (with 50 brands) for five years – branding, product development and marketing copywriting. This experience led to me creating my own company, Get Branded Press, which is all about beauty, branding and books.

Having spoken to women for years about beauty, with focus on taking care of their skin and embracing their natural beauty, I wrote the book *Sexy, Fit & Fab at Any Age!* followed up by *Sexy, Fit & Fab Sirens* (with 24 contributing authors) – in which I asked Karla to share her story of success in the beauty industry. Karla's story is very inspiring and many women and skin care experts can relate to it, *"Success is when passion meets money."* As Karla has been contributing her writings for years in the beauty industry, I asked her what her next step was in sharing her story and knowledge on a bigger scale. She shared that she'd actually been writing content for a beauty book, *Your Esthetics Coach.*

Karla diligently went to work writing her manuscript, all while continuing to build and grow her successful skin care company. It has been so exciting to help Karla bring *Your Esthetics Coach* book and brand to life!

I am so inspired by Karla's work ethic, an attitude of excellence in all she does, and I know that other Estheticians and beauty experts will take away so much from this book, *Your Esthetics Coach*. I'm grateful to have worked with Karla, and this manual is like taking Karla home with you – teaching you everything you will need to know about how to become a successful Esthetician behind the chair. Karla's humor makes learning fun, as she shares her "Lessons" that are sprinkled throughout this book, teaching you everything you need to know about the skin, skin conditions and how to treat them, as well as how to connect with and educate your clients on their skin. In this day and age, everyone wants to look and feel younger, and Karla's anti-aging tips will empower you to make a measurable difference in your clients' skin. I challenge you to continue your skin care education and take your career to the next level.

Live the life of your dreams and follow your passion!

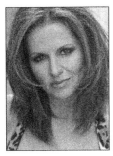 **SUSIE AUGUSTIN** is the bestselling author of *Sexy, Fit & Fab at Any Age!*, *Sexy, Fit & Fab Sirens*, and upcoming *Sexy, Fit & Fab Beauty Secrets*. Her writing, speaking and publishing have garnered her Awards and Nominations. She is a Beauty & Branding Expert and has worked with some of the world's top rated beauty companies. Susie is committed to helping women increase their self-confidence and improve their body image through exploring their inner and outer beauty, inspiring them to develop their essences, exude confidence, embrace their true selves and feel extraordinary. To help others pursue their dreams and brand themselves through their writing, Susie wrote *Writing to Wow! Book Writing Workbook* and created Get Branded Press, offering editing, ghostwriting and publishing. Her mission is *Dream it. Write it. Brand it.* *www.SexyFitFab.com*

Introduction

As a licensed Cosmetologist with an emphasis on Esthetics for over three decades, I have had the blessing of working with all aspects of the business of beauty and skin care. From being an Educator my entire career and having taught thousands of Estheticians over the years, I have often been asked to write a book to share my knowledge. My goal with this book is to guide, share, and mentor you in most aspects of your esthetics business and to empower you to be the best skin care expert within.

I am often asked, "How did you get here? What's your secret to success?" Most successful people can most likely contribute their success to a life event, a circumstance, a person or people, or an opportunity. I view mine as a lifetime of events, a lifetime of circumstances, a lifetime of people, and a lifetime of amazing opportunities.

My passion to be an Esthetician started at a very early age, long before anyone could even pronounce the word "Esthetician", let alone understand what we did. My tireless passion for our craft has provided me with many blessed opportunities and I have worked with some of the greats in the esthetics industry. Without my mentors, I wouldn't have experienced my success or have the knowledge that I have. In addition, I have been a perpetual student of this ever-changing and evolving industry of ours.

It all started when I was a very little girl around the age of five. I remember being mesmerized by my very girlie Grandma Lou's beautiful fragrance bottles and high end jars of creams and bottles of lotions in her bathroom. You see, I was destined to be in the beauty industry, I just didn't know it yet. As a senior in high school, I was unsure of what my future was going to bring. I knew that the conventional college path wasn't calling me. It was then, in a long line of mentors throughout my life, that my high school guidance teacher suggested cosmetology school. The light bulb went on, and for the first time I felt the excitement and gained the passion that I have had for this industry for over 33 years. Off I went to beauty school moving far away from my home. So excited that I didn't think through any of the details such as how I was going to live, eat, pay for rent, etc. Much as to how I still live my life. I figure that stuff out as I go. I have always believed that money follows passion. Passion rarely follows money. I went on and graduated the top of my class and received a scholarship for the first Advanced Esthetic Post Graduate Training Institute in Chicago to specialize in skin care. It was there that I met a mentor of a lifetime. He taught me everything there was to know. He is still to this day coined as "the pioneer of esthetics". He believed in me and shortly after with a lot of tenacity and begging, I began to work for his company as the Director of Training at age 24. This then put me on the fast track to meet several more key people, hold many executive positions, and meet many more mentors.

Fast forward to now, reflectively, it is all of those experiences, every one of them, good and bad, that has placed me right here today and where I will be tomorrow and the next day. My unwavering role in this was that I always have integrity, tenacity, and exceptional work ethic, and overall, was a kind, considerate, compassionate person.

I have now reached what I call my "sweet spot of success". It is when passion *finally* meets money. It all has gone full circle and everything now makes perfect sense. I have learned that success isn't always about money. It is about loving what you do and also becoming financially successful doing it.

Your Esthetics Coach will teach you the 6 Steps to becoming a successful Esthetician behind the chair. We'll take a look at all the tools in your toolbox, understanding how each is to be utilized, as well as what precautions should be taken. The education you obtain will help take you to the next level. You will learn how to conduct a skin analysis, and gain valuable tips on how to perform a client consultation.

Learn how to guide your clients in making smart choices in skin care, yielding powerful results.

You will learn how and why the skin functions, behaves and reacts the way it does. Understanding skin conditions and how to treat them will build trust with your clientele. Educating them on skin care products, ingredients, and making a measurable difference in the quality of their skin will help you to increase your product sales and services, helping you to increase your income.

Make yourself stand out by learning beneficial extraction tips and techniques that you can start today. Your enthusiasm for listening and connecting with your clients, as well as mastering the facial massage, will build long lasting relationships with your clients. With the education you acquire from *Your Esthetics Coach*, you can take on a leadership role in your community, partnering up with other businesses in ways that will help grow your business.

My hope is that this book will inspire you to follow your passion and make an impact in the beauty industry… by continuing to educate and empower yourself, having the confidence to make a difference in your clients' skin and lives.

BEGINNER'S
BASICS

> "I get really excited when I think of the potential that we have as Estheticians to have an impact on people's lives."
>
> *Karla Keene, L.E.*

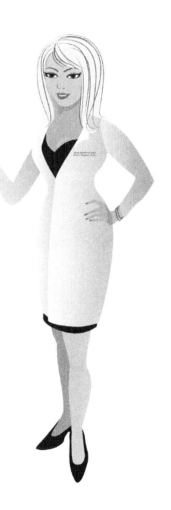

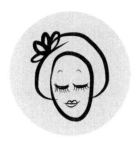

An Esthetician's Scope of Practice

Estheticians are finally being acknowledged as true professionals that have the ability to change the way someone's skin behaves, appears, and ages! Today we can do so much more than just "sprinkle, pour, rub, or massage" lotions and potions to "beautify" the skin. With the right education and the right "tools" in our tool box (products and equipment), we can make a difference in how our clients feel about themselves – physically, emotionally and psychologically. How powerful! What a tremendous and gratifying field of work we are in.

The skin care industry is a rapidly growing and exciting industry to be a part of. As the industry expands, the need for highly trained Estheticians is at an all-time high. It takes a lot of hard work, time, education and training, with the right "tableside manner" to be successful in this extremely competitive industry. I want to explore all of these elements throughout the book and share some lessons and pearls of wisdom that can help put you on the fast track to success.

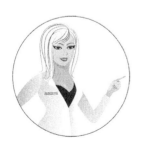

LESSON #1

"The professional skin care market is shifting. The majority of facial clients are seeking professional advice and requesting services and products that will yield results!"

I will coach you throughout this book on the right recipes for results. It all starts there! Most clients today want the money that they spend on their skin to be commensurate with the results that they see. In other words, **they will spend if we deliver!** We rarely experience the dedicated client (who invests in facials on a regular basis), who is just looking to relax and want what I call the "fluff & buff, feel good facial". I tend to see more of this type of facial at a resort, destination spa, or cruise ships where the goal is to relax. One thing we know for sure. Today's savvy client **knows more** and **wants more** and we need to be able to deliver!

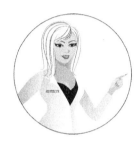

LESSON #2
"As skin care providers, we must do our clients no harm. This is the basis for infection prevention and control."

Sanitation/Infection Control Regulations

Safety first is of the utmost importance for you and for your clients. We must practice by OSHA and state guidelines. Safety precautions and sanitation are vital to your success. Hand washing and hand sterilizing before and after every client, and when necessary throughout the service, is paramount. Glove wearing with extractions is always necessary. As a skin care specialist, be especially careful in your practice against infection if you have clients with viruses, because they can spread to you or other clients by indirect as well as direct contact.

What Can You Expect to Make Behind the Chair?

I am often asked what Estheticians can potentially earn working behind the chair. There are so many variables to this answer. The potential is endless, albeit, it takes a lot of knowledge, endurance, patience, hard work and time to build your business. I know Estheticians who have all of the above, who easily make six figure incomes behind the chair. According to Indeed.com, the average salary (at the time of writing this book) for an Esthetician is $40,000 per year. However, as clearly indicated in the graph below, that number is growing every year. An Esthetician's income will vary based on many different factors such as location, self-employed or employed, if paid on commission or salary, the level of education, and how many years in practice.

National Salary Trend from Indeed.com
– Esthetician

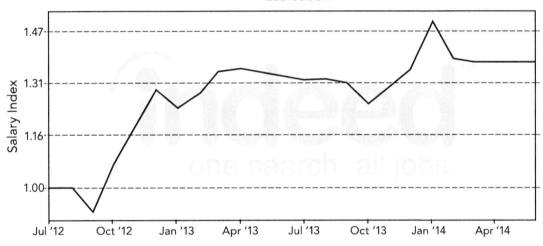

http://www.indeed.com/salary/Esthetician.html

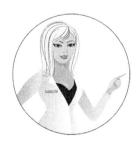

LESSON #3

"Set your own goals on how much you want to make, and then design a plan on how to make it! The sky is the limit!"

Our Scope of Practice... What We Can and Cannot Do

According to Wikipedia, "Estheticians (sometimes referred to as Aestheticians) are licensed professionals who are experts in maintaining and improving a healthy epidermis. An Esthetician's general scope of practice is limited to the epidermis (the outer layer of skin)."

Within our scope of practice we can help to prevent, control, and correct most of the unwanted esthetic conditions that your clients experience.

We also must clearly understand what our limitations are as skin care providers. It is important that we don't diagnose medical skin conditions nor make any promises to treat them. What may appear to be a skin disease and/or disorder needs to be referred to a dermatologist or other medical professional for diagnosis and treatment.

Understand Your State Regulations

The Scope of Practice for Estheticians is governed by the each individual state, and they can change often and quickly. Each state's regulations vary when it comes to what and where services can be performed and by whom, and with what equipment and products. It is important that you fully understand the scope of practice for Estheticians within the state that you are practicing in, and review it often. Everything from room setup regulations, linens, tools, products, and more can be different from state to state.

The 6 Simple Steps to Success

have always said that success can mean many different things to different Estheticians. What is driving you? Do you have a passion for skin care? Is it money? Or both? The latter is where we see the most success.

Money means success and success means money, for most. My idea of success is when passion meets money. I have determined that there are *6 Steps to Becoming a Successful Esthetician Behind the Chair*, and in this order.

1. You Must Continue to Educate Yourself

In order to sell yourself, your products and your services, you have to have the confidence to do so. **Confidence begins with EDUCATION!** We can never stop learning and growing, particularly in such a fluid, ever-growing industry as ours. Invest time in your career by taking all relevant and interesting classes that you can attend via your product or equipment manufacturers, associations, trade shows, and the like. We have to stay ahead of the curve, especially since our clients are much more skin savvy, educated and interested than ever before.

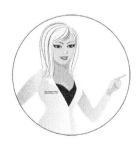

LESSON #4
"First, we must do what we love and love what we do!"

2. Empower Yourself to be the Expert

Become an expert at what you do! What, if anything, may be holding you back from becoming the best Esthetician that you can be? Aspire to be the go-to skin care expert in your immediate area. This can take some time, diligence and a lot of hard work.

First, to succeed, we have to be the best at what we do. Our clients are looking to us for expert advice. When they visit a licensed skin care professional such as ourselves, they assume that we know more than the counter girls at the big box retail stores. We do! We are the ones that have gone through formal training and are licensed to provide clients with the quality, efficacy, safety and results that they deserve. We are still losing a large percentage of retail sales to non-licensed counter staff at the retail level. We must learn what it is that we need to do to educate our clients enough to trust us, and to only buy from us as professionals.

We do this by having a thorough, comprehensive understanding of all of our products and equipment. Learn everything there is to know about the products you are recommending including price, benefits, usage and ingredients. Do you personally use the products that you sell? How can you sell what you don't know or are not familiar with? We need to know and believe in what we are offering, or it could translate negatively onto our clients.

Remember...

 Your clients have come to you because they need or want what you have.

 They want and expect your expert advice about their skin.

 Don't do them a disservice. Your clients deserve:

- The best overall experience
- The best consultation
- A thorough skin analysis
- A detailed treatment plan
- A recommended home care regimen
- The results that they are looking for
- To know what they need and how often they need it

Do you consider yourself to be an expert in skin care? _____

If you answered no, what steps are you going to take to become one?

_____

_____

_____

_____

In this highly competitive industry that we work in, in order to be successful, we need to be an expert to stand out amongst the competitors. Education is the key to do just that!

3. Educate Your Clients:
Education = Sales = More Income

Use what you know and know what you use! Educating your clients always generates sales, both in services and in retail products. Why? Because you establish a level of trust and credibility with your clients when you educate them, which in turn makes them feel confident and comfortable with making a buying decision.

4. Experience the Benefits of Increased Product and Service Sales

When you educate your clients and sell more products and services, as a result, everybody wins. The client benefits with more youthful skin; you increase your sales and become more successful!

Let's talk about the not-so-comfortable word "selling". It can be a very big contributing factor to your success, or lack of. Many of us Estheticians are very nurturing by nature; hence, we don't like to think of ourselves as "sales people". If you think about it, we sell ourselves every day. I am going to challenge you to change the way that you think about selling. I want you to see it as educating the client.

EDUCATION = SALES. ALWAYS.

I will provide many sales tips throughout this book on ways to increase your income through suggestive selling, creating treatment plans, and more!

A couple of things to think about…

- If you haven't made selling a focus or part of your strategy to build your business yet, *start now!* This is your business, or your business within a business, even if you work for others. **All businesses require sales to thrive, including yours.**
- You are responsible for creating your income… you are in control of your success! The sky is the limit!

List your ideas, strategies, and goals to increase your sales abilities and to reach new monetary goals:

_____
_____
_____
_____
_____
_____
_____

5. As a Result, You Make More Money

It is no secret that we feel rewarded when we make money doing what we love. This formula is quite simple and has a domino effect on our business.

> # When we make more money = we are happier and more positive at work = when we are happy at work we tend to have better job satisfaction and longevity.

6. Most Importantly, You Increase Your Client Retention

Building a loyal book of business can take time and lots of hard work. It is easier to retain an existing customer than it is to aquire new ones. Client retention comes from happy, satisfied clients who see results. These are the clients who are most likely to continue to spend money with you and refer potential new clients to you.

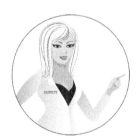

LESSON #5

"Remember, your clients are buying their skin care products somewhere. It might as well be with you!"

How Important are Results?

I would like to focus, again, on the importance of achieving your clients' goals and seeing RESULTS. Ultimately, that is what brings our clients back and is a mandatory piece to achieving success. There are many spokes to the wheel to delivering results, which include having the proper techniques, protocols, products, and equipment, which offer an amazing overall client "experience".

So, in a nutshell...when we deliver results, we become more trusted by our clients, they tend to refer more clients to us, we build our business, and we make more money! Sound like a plan? If you bring the passion, it is my goal to provide you not just information on "how to become successful", but a plan on "how to make money" doing it! That is what I call the "sweet spot"- making money at what you love to do! One thing that I've learned over the course of my career is that money follows passion...passion rarely follows money. So stay passionate and keep learning. Do what you love and love what you do! The money part inevitably follows.

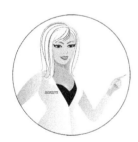

LESSON #6
"Success is when passion meets money."

The Look and Voice of Authority

A significant portion of your clients' reaction to your overall authority is based on non-verbal communication. Do you appear polished and carry yourself with confidence? You want to radiate confidence and professional knowledge. Be ready for your day. After all, we are in the beauty business! Hair should be clean and done, nails to be clean and short, skin to be healthy and clear, and your makeup to be fresh (and refreshed when needed). Always look your best!

Did you know that the largest percentage of a client's reaction to your recommendations for services and home care products will be based upon your outward appearance (non-verbal communication)? And that a very small percentage will be based on the words you use and technical ability (verbal communication)?

Do you look in the mirror at yourself before you go to work?

_____

_____

What do you see?

_____

_____

List some of the ways you could improve your look of authority.

_____

_____

_____

_____

_____

_____

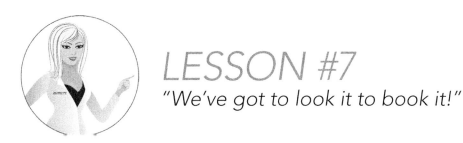

LESSON #7
"We've got to look it to book it!"

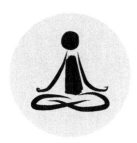

Back to Basics...
The Anatomy &
Physiology of the Skin

Ok, let's go back to the very beginning for a minute. Back to the very basics of what we do. The very fundamental *Anatomy & Physiology of the Skin 101*. What do we really need to understand? Clearly, we must understand the dynamics and functions of the skin before we can expect to create a skin wellness plan for our clients. How does it work? How can we influence change with our products and services? How does the skin absorb? How does the skin respond to certain ingredients and why?

To know this information and more helps us to understand how we can influence the skin from the inside out and from the outside in. We can change the way people feel about their skin through the combination of understanding how the skin works, along with knowing what ingredients and products can influence positive changes in their skin.

Just the Facts. Our Skin is...
- Like a window to our internal health
- An amazing self-healing, self-regenerating organ
- Resilient, yet responds well to attention
- One of the most exposed, abused organs of the body, yet least cared for

Beautiful, healthy skin is determined by the health of the structure and proper function of the constituents within the skin. To maintain beautiful skin, and to slow the rate at which it ages, the structures and functions of the skin must be modified, nurtured, supplemented and protected. In order to do so, it's important to know as much as you can about the skin's basic anatomy and physiology.

What is the Skin Made Of?
- The skin is the largest organ in the body, comprising about 15% of the body weight.
- In adults, the skin covers an area of about 2 square meters, and weighs 4.5 to 5 kg.
- It ranges in thickness from 0.5 to 4.0 mm, depending on the area of the body.
- The total skin surface of an adult ranges from 12 to 20 square feet.
- The skin is made up of approximately 70% water, 25% protein and 2% lipids.

The Main Functions of the Skin

Sometimes we look at our skin from a vanity perspective only. And that caring for our skin is directly related only to how we look, and how our skin ages. Our skin is actually created for physiological reasons first. Hence, it is so important to educate ourselves and our clients on the need for preventative skin care. The skin needs to function normally and in a healthy manner, in order for it to look healthy and youthful on the outside. Take a look at some of the really important physiological functions that our skin was designed to do.

- **Skin Shields the Body** – The skin provides a physical shield that protects the underlying physiology from physical harm, bacterial infection, water loss, and more. Think of the skin as armor. Without the function of a strong armor, we leave our bodies and skin vulnerable to skin disorders, diseases, and premature aging. We need to work at always keeping our skin healthy, strong, and resilient.

THE SKIN

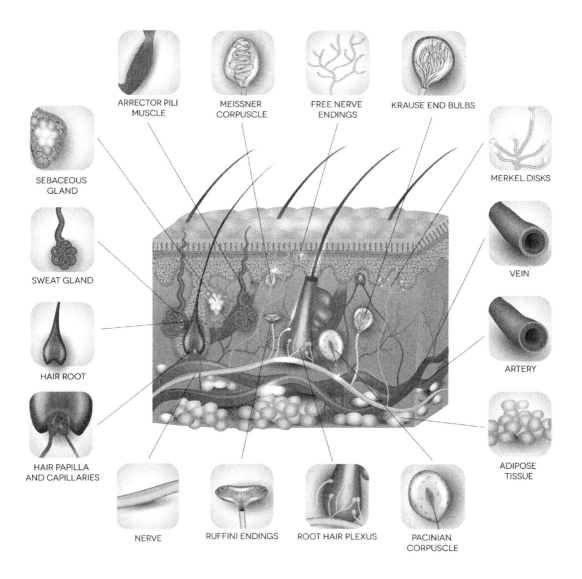

ARRECTOR PILI MUSCLE

MEISSNER CORPUSCLE

FREE NERVE ENDINGS

KRAUSE END BULBS

SEBACEOUS GLAND

MERKEL DISKS

SWEAT GLAND

VEIN

HAIR ROOT

ARTERY

HAIR PAPILLA AND CAPILLARIES

ADIPOSE TISSUE

NERVE

RUFFINI ENDINGS

ROOT HAIR PLEXUS

PACINIAN CORPUSCLE

- **Provides Hot/Cold Temperature Regulation** – Vascular structures in the skin are able to vasodilate and vasoconstrict under the influence of our nervous system.
  — Vasodilation brings more blood to the surface of the body.
     Stimulation also kicks in the skin's self-regenerating mechanisms, increases water and oil production, increases cellular proliferation.
  — Vasoconstriction reduces blood flow.
     Sedation slows down the skin's metabolism, reduces inflammation.

- **Sensory Control** – Millions of nerve endings in the skin detect our interaction with external factors.

- **Elimination** – Waste products such as urea and lactic acid are excreted when we sweat, to detoxify the skin and body.

- **Resistance** – The epidermis fends off foreign aggressors like environmental factors, exposure to harmful elements, and more.

- **Blood Tank** – The dermis of the skin houses extensive complexes of blood vessels that carry 8 to 10% of the total blood movement.

Notes:

_____

_____

_____

_____

_____

_____

_____

_____

_____

_____

_____

_____

_____

_____

_____

The Skin Consists of Two Layers – the Epidermis and the Dermis

Structure of the Epidermis

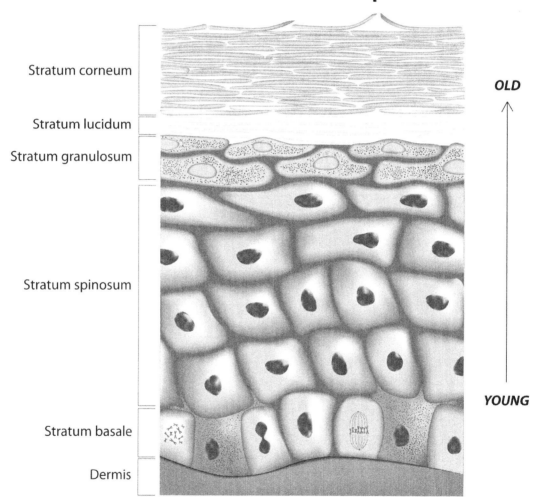

Stratum corneum

Stratum lucidum

Stratum granulosum

Stratum spinosum

Stratum basale

Dermis

OLD

YOUNG

Epidermis

The epidermis is the outermost layer of the skin. It is categorized into five distinct layers. The total depth of the epidermis is usually about 0.5 to 1 mm.

There are Four Cell Types Present in the Epidermis:

- **Keratinocytes**

  These cells make the protein called keratin, and are the prime kind of cells found in the epidermis.

  Keratinocytes produce keratin, which is a protein that toughens and waterproofs the skin.

  — They are found at the lowermost portion of the epidermis and divide rapidly.

  — As they mature, keratinocytes lose water, flatten out and move upward. Eventually, at the end of their life cycle (28-30 days), they reach the surface of the epidermis called stratum corneum.

- **Melanocytes**

  These cells produce melanin, a pigment that is responsible for skin color.

- **Langerhans**

  These cells are macrophages that interact with white blood cells during an immune response.

  — They can prevent unwanted external substances from penetrating the skin.

- **Merkel Cells**

  These cells are found deep in the epidermis at the epidermal-dermal boundary.

  — They, in connection with nerve endings, serve a sensory function.

There are Five Layers to the Epidermis:
- The **stratum corneum** contains many layers of dead keratinocytes. The outermost layers are constantly sloughing.
- The **stratum lucidum** layer is usually apparent only in thick skin.
- The **stratum granulosum** contains layers of cells held together by desmosomes. These cells provide the growth of keratin in the upper layers of the epidermis, and bind dead cells together.
- The **stratum spinosum** contains cells connected by desmosomes. These cells are moderately active in mitosis/division.
- The **stratum basale** contains cells actively dividing by mitosis, to produce cells that migrate to the surface of the skin.

The epidermis can be very resilient and resistive depending on the condition. Most skin care treatments and products have the greatest or direct impact on this layer of skin. The desired result for this layer is to be free of imperfections, feel soft to the touch, have integrity, and be pliable and flexible.

Dermis

The middle level of the skin, the dermis, consists of various connective tissues. As a connective tissue, it contains fibroblasts and macrophages along with collagen, elastic, hyaluronic acid and fibers. The structure provides strength, extensibility (the ability to be stretched), and elasticity (the ability to return to its original form).

The Dermis Consists of Two Layers:
- The **papillary layer** is a thin, outer layer with tiny protrusions called dermal papillae that move into the epidermis.
- The **reticular layer** is a thick layer, below the papillary layer, that makes up most of the dermis.

The dermis is located between the epidermis and subcutaneous tissue.
  — It is the thickest of the skin layers.
  — Both collagen and elastin are produced here and are important skin proteins; and as we know, collagen is responsible for the structural support and elastin for the resilience of the skin.
  — The key type of cells in the dermis are fibroblasts, which create collagen and elastin.
- The dermis also contains capillaries and lymph nodes.
  — These are important for oxygenating, nourishing, and protecting the skin.
- The dermis contains sebaceous glands, sweat glands, and hair follicles.
  — Sebaceous glands are of great importance for skin as they produce sebum, an oily protective substance that lubricates and waterproofs the skin.
- The dermis also contains glycosaminoglycans – these are moisture-binding molecules that provide moisture to the epidermis.

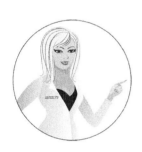

LESSON #8

"The desired goal for the dermal layer is to maintain or increase metabolism, increase cellular proliferation, encourage new collagen growth, increase glandular activity and increase blood flow."

Hypodermis

The hypodermis (subcutaneous layer) lies between the dermis and underlying tissues and organs.

- It consists of mostly adipose (fat) tissue.
- Subcutaneous fat acts as a shock absorber to protect the skin from trauma.
- Is a great heat insulator, protecting the skin's structure from cold.
- The loss of subcutaneous tissue, often occurring with age, leads to facial hollowing.

More About the Skin

The following accessory organs are also found within the skin:

- Hairs arise and emerge from the skin.
- Sudoriferous (sweat) glands secrete sweat. Sweat consists of water with various salts and other substances.

There are Four Kinds of Sudoriferous Glands:

- **Eccrine Glands** occur under most skin surfaces and secrete a watery solution through pores, which serve to cool the skin as it evaporates. There are 2.5 to 3 million eccrine sweat glands in the skin.
- **Apocrine Glands** occur under skin surfaces of the armpits and pubic regions and, beginning with puberty, secrete a solution in response to stress. The solution, more viscous than that secreted by eccrine glands, is secreted into hair follicles.
- **Ceruminous Glands** secrete cerumen (earwax) into the external ear canal. Wax helps to impede the entrance of foreign bodies.
- **Sebaceous (oil) Glands** secrete sebum, an oily substance, into hair follicles or sometimes through skin surface pores.
  — Sebum also contributes to the lipids and fatty acids within the moisture barrier.
  — Sebum inhibits bacterial growth and helps prevent drying of the skin.
  — An accumulation of sebum in the duct of a sebaceous gland produces whiteheads, blackheads (if the sebum oxidizes), and acne (if the sebum becomes infected by bacteria).

NMF (Natural Moisture Factor)

The combination of the eccrine gland secreting water and the sebaceous gland secreting oil creates our *Natural Moisture Factor.*

- The Eccrine gland is responsible to hydrate the stratum corneum layer of the epidermis while the sebaceous gland provides the oil to "lock in" the moisture.
- This prevents Trans Epidermal Water Loss (TEWL).

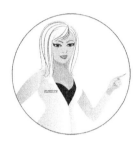

LESSON #9

"The sudoriferous (sweat) glands in our skin secrete 10% of all of the body's waste through the follicles in our skin. Our skin is literally a dumping ground."

What happens to these important functions through the intrinsic (natural) aging process?

- They begin to slow down just like all of the other mechanisms within the skin.
- They produce less water and oil.

What does this mean to the overall health of the skin?

What can we do through topical applications of products to improve?

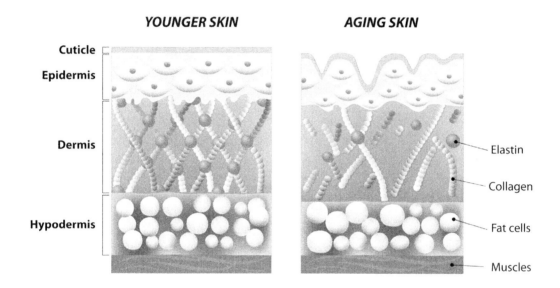

YOUNGER SKIN   **AGING SKIN**

Cuticle
Epidermis

Dermis — Elastin

— Collagen

Hypodermis — Fat cells

— Muscles

Pores

The skin cells that line the pore (keratinocytes) are continuously shed, just like the cells of the epidermis at the top of the skin.

- The keratinocytes being shed from the lining of the pore can mix with sebum and clog the pore. This is the precursor to acne.
- If oil and debris build up inside the pores, or if tissue surrounding the pore becomes inflamed, pores may appear larger.

*Remember…*the aging process of the skin begins the minute we are born.

It has been thought that we lose 1% of the collagen in our skin for every year that we are alive. We absolutely can preserve our skin health through comprehensive maintenance skin care. Just like all other organs, the skin also slows down as we age. Therefore, we need to supplement the skin as it matures, just as we do for the rest of our bodies.

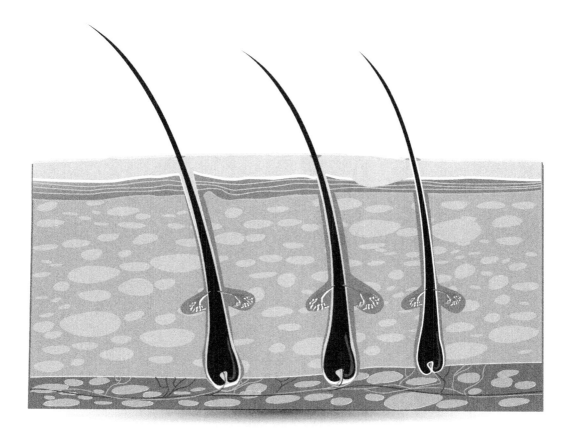

UNDERSTANDING THE TOOLS OF OUR TRADE...
THEIR USAGE & BENEFITS

"As part of our collection of tools, we have so many modalities that can play a tremendous role in the achievement of clear, healthy skin for our clients. Let's examine our professional-use esthetic equipment and products."

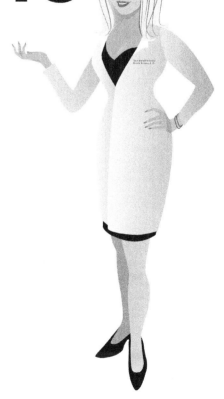

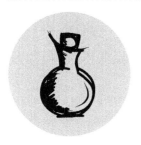

Products/Ingredients

I could write an entire book on this topic as it my true passion and has been a big part of my career. I have spent my entire career learning, understanding, and teaching about products and ingredients. This is a very fluid area of our industry, as we see so much exciting growth and new information about topical skin care ingredients on a regular basis. You can never stop learning! But we also have to be very cognizant that there is also a lot of media hype on products and ingredients that are not supported by science. We have to be able to differentiate fads vs. trends, credible information vs. biased opinions, marketing vs. realistic expectations, and the like. There are also many other factors that need to be taken into consideration when attempting to choose a healthy, results-driven product, such as the grade of ingredients, percentages of the performing ingredients within the formula, pH, vehicles, molecular size, and more! Let's take a closer look…

List here why you think consumers make the choices that they do when choosing to purchase their skin care products.

_____
_____
_____
_____
_____
_____
_____
_____
_____
_____
_____
_____
_____
_____

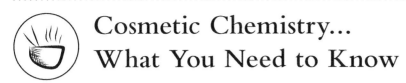

Cosmetic Chemistry...
What You Need to Know

One thing I do know is that not all products can be created equally. From one manufacturer to another, they can differ drastically, albeit, may physically look the same, as well as have similar ingredient decks. We can tell a little bit more about a product by its ingredient list yet, there is much speculation or little transparency as to the full meaning of the label, as our FDA only mandates a few things for us to understand via cosmetic packaging. Much of the rest of the labeling is designed by the manufacturer to increase the perceived value to prompt the consumer to buy, along with beautiful packaging, fragrances, and impressive marketing materials. I will discuss some of these topics in this chapter to further inform you of what to look for and what to be aware of, so that we can properly educate our clients and not perpetuate more misinformation.

How to Really Interpret an Ingredient List

Typically, when we as professionals as well as consumers look at an ingredient list, we simply are seeking ingredients that we are aware of, to teach us more about the value or intended use of the product. One of the few mandates that we have by the FDA to interpret the label, is the order of which the ingredients are listed. They should be listed in order of predominance in a descending order. Any ingredient that is below a volume of .1% does not have to be listed at all, unless it is an over the counter monographed drug. On the other hand, I have seen where manufacturers do what I call "load the deck", where they load the ingredient list with everything under the sun to also increase the perceived value of the product when, in fact, they may contain such small percentages that those ingredients may not impact the way that the product works, if at all. This is a "trick" that many manufacturers can easily use to make that product seem to offer more than what it can, or does.

I have always taught that we should take a closer look at the first 5 to 8 ingredients on the list. These ingredients typically will make up the majority of what is in the bottle or jar. If you discover that there are lots of chemicals you can't pronounce, preservatives, colorants, fragrances, filler materials (i.e. waxes, petrochemicals, etc.) in the top 5 to 8 ingredients, this usually indicates that this may not be the healthiest product, and/or may not be results-driven, and more importantly, may be harmful. On the other hand, if you are seeing high volumes of corrective ingredients such as retinols, alpha hydroxyl acids, beta hydroxyl acids, antioxidants and the like, there is a good chance that these products are more of a performing type of product.

I have always thought that it is fair to say that we can divide products into two categories (both professional and retail), depending on the myriad of reasons women and men buy/need personal care products.

1. **Cosmetic** – Feel good/smell good product, nurturing, spa-like, great esoteric values (smell and feel good) yet, not necessarily corrective in nature.
2. **Corrective** – Therapeutic, high performance, results-driven, changes the way the skin looks and feels, and is considered more serious skin care for those looking to improve their unwanted conditions.

I think it is also fair to say that to really understand a product, we must first look at the entire makeup of the product. It is in my opinion, that there are six important areas to take into consideration when determining if a product is safe and/or effective.

The 6 Spokes to the Wheel of a Safe, Results-Driven Product

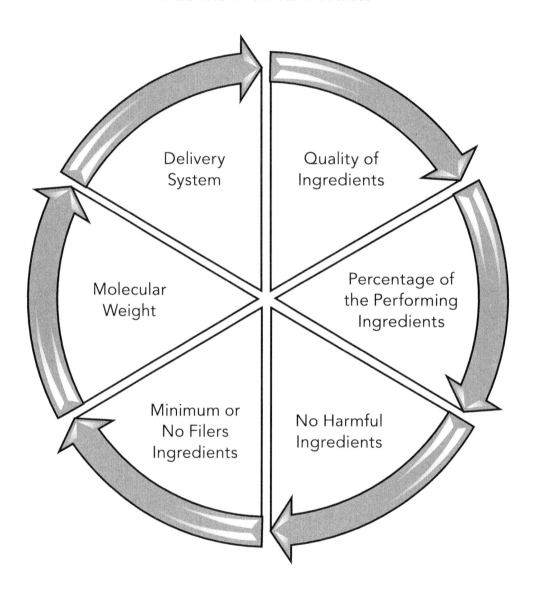

1. Quality of Ingredients.

The quality of the ingredients used is critical criteria to consider when creating a safe product. Also, we see much less allergic type of adverse reactions to a higher quality of these ingredients.

2. Percentage of the Performing Ingredients.

There has to be enough of the performing ingredient to actually see results.

3. Does it Contain Harmful Ingredients?

The addition of harmful ingredients can negate the positive outcome of the healthy ingredients. Not to mention the harmful effects of the individual ingredients.

4. Does it Contain High Levels of Several Filler Materials?

Filler ingredients are often used to create the majority or bulk of the ingredients within the ingredient list to create an inexpensive product, whereas the motive is profit and not productivity/results.

5. What is the Molecular Weight?

We need to be aware that in order for most ingredients to work synergistically within the skin, they must need to be absorbed, albeit, depends on the intended use of the ingredient. For example, if the ingredient is used as a lubricant to soften the texture of the skin, a larger molecular weight may be more appropriate.

6. What is the Product's Delivery System (if any)?

Maximum absorption is critical when needing the skin to respond.

Additionally, there are other issues that we need to consider. In the past and present, there are terms that we hear a lot of in skin care, such as "cosmeceuticals" or "nutricosmetics". What do these terms mean? These are strictly marketing tactics that manufacturers use loosely… when they should be limited to being used as a description/differentiator when defining those cosmetic products with biologically active ingredients, supported by science, purporting to have extraordinary benefits; albeit, the terms are not recognized by the FDA. These terms are often used in cosmetic advertising, and may be misleading to the consumer.

According to the United States Food and Drug Administration (FDA), the Food, Drug, and Cosmetic Act *"does not recognize any such category as "cosmeceuticals." A product can be a drug, a cosmetic, or a combination of both, but the term "cosmeceutical" has no meaning under the law"*.

These terms have now been "watered down" in the marketplace, now used widely for marketing purposes, having very little merit, hoping to give a product line "credibility", or to give a perception of higher quality. They are losing their steam. Rather than getting caught up in the latest fads and terms, again, I differentiate good vs. bad, effective vs. non-effective, as either "cosmetic" or "corrective".

Corrective type products have been around the dermatologic and plastic surgery market for quite some time. Also, many of these types of performance-based products are now made available in an over-the-counter preparation that can be prescribed by licensed professionals like yourself.

What is Safe and What Isn't?

Cosmetic technology has advanced exponentially. Dermatological research suggests that the bioactive ingredients used in skin care products today do indeed have benefits beyond the traditional moisturizer (e.g., Chen et al., 2005[1]; Zettersten, Ghadially, Feingold, Crumrine, & Elias, 1997[2])

However, there are still many cosmetic ingredients that are proven to be unhealthy, unsafe, and potentially dangerous. The lenient regulatory oversight for this $35 plus billion dollar industry leads to companies routinely marketing products with ingredients that are poorly studied, not studied at all, or worse, known to pose potentially serious health risks. Because much of the testing is voluntary and controlled by the manufacturers, many ingredients in cosmetic products are not safety tested at all. I last read that 89% of 10,500 ingredients used in personal care products have not been evaluated for safety by the CIR (Cosmetic Ingredient Review), the FDA, nor any other publicly accountable institution. One of every 100 products on the market contain ingredients certified by government authorities as known or probable human carcinogens, including shampoos, conditioners, creams, lotions, makeup foundations, moisturizers, and lip balms. An astonishing one-third of all products contain one or more ingredients classified as possible human carcinogens. There are no federal standards for ingredient purity. While it seems likely that some companies purchase or manufacture refined, purified ingredients, it is equally likely that many do not. Consumers and government health officials have no way to know.

Quality Matters!
What We Put on Our Skin...Gets in Our Skin!

It has been well documented as of recent that a large percentage of what we put on our skin gets in our skin within seconds. Should we be concerned with quality and safety? Yes! We are what we use on our skin!

Way back when, a 1970 study of skin on skin absorption of nine organic chemicals demonstrated the body's capacity to absorb up to 43% of the applied dose over a 5 day period. Today, with new micronization techniques, new ingredients, etc., we know even more to validate that need to be concerned with the quality of what we are recommending to our clients. Many of these chemicals are being absorbed through the skin when applying creams, lotions, deodorants and hair dyes, ingested when used in toothpastes, mouthwashes and lipsticks, and inhaled with aerosol sprays for hair care and spray deodorants. Think about when we use cosmetic products on a daily basis applying small quantities of all types of synthetic chemicals to our bodies, what a cumulative effect this must have on not just our skin, but our bodies and health!

The 4 Criteria for Evaluating Skin Care Products

Criteria to determine whether they are "body-friendly" and effective or not.
1. Toxicity
2. Occlusivity
3. Comedogenicity
4. Effectiveness

1. Toxicity

Toxicity of skin care ingredients may be divided into three distinct categories:

1) **Carcinogenic**
   Refers to ingredients that have been proven to contribute to cancer in our bodies through absorption.

2) **Endocrine-Disrupting**
   Refers to chemicals that disturb the body's hormonal balance, and may interfere with its ability to function normally. Endocrine disruptors may also be carcinogenic.

3) **Allergenic**
   Consumers may have allergic reactions or develop contact dermatitis (itching, redness, rash, etc.) more easily with these types of ingredients over others.

Of the enormous list of cosmetic ingredients, relatively few individually pose extreme high risk, but many people use a large amount of personal care products every day. It may be that these risks are cumulative, or that some ingredients don't react well with others and create toxic combinations, known as synergistic toxicity.

A bit of a side note about preservatives. I am a strong proponent against the use of parabens in skin care. There is enough data on the fence for me to choose to not formulate with or to use on myself personally. We will discuss this in more detail under the "Harmful Cosmetic Ingredients" section of this book. By their very nature, preservatives are toxic. However, we must keep in mind that percentage, quality, and type all play a part of that statement.

2. Occlusivity

The skin is the body's largest organ. We often refer to the skin "needing to breathe". The "breathing" of the skin refers to the skin's ability to rid itself of toxins and chemicals through excretion (perspiration). Lotions and ointment type ingredients/products that occlude this exchange may initially soften the skin by keeping moisture from escaping, but long term use of occlusive products/ingredients could cause comedogenicity or onset of acne, irritation, etc., actually inhibiting the overall health of the skin. We can also tout the benefits of occasional use of occlusive products, in that they help to lock in the skin's Natural Moisture Factor.

3. Comedogenicity

Comedogenicity refers to the ability of an ingredient to get into the skin's pores and clog them. The word "comedo" is the medical term for blackhead, so comedo + genic means "friendly to blackheads." There are many factors to take into consideration when determining if a finished product is comedogenic.
1. Percentage of the comedogenic ingredient within the formula.
2. Number of comedogenic ingredients within the same formula.
3. Time on tissue. The length of time the product is left on the skin.

Here are what I call the "Top Eight" highly comedogenic ingredients used in skin care products to watch out for:
- Acetyl Lanolin Alcohol
- Butyl Stearate
- Isopropyl Myristate
- Octyl Palmitate
- Flax Oil
- Isocetyl Stearate
- Myristal Myristate
- Castor Oil

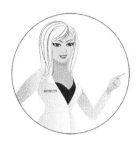

LESSON #10

"The important thing is to look at positioning in the ingredient list. Hint: If a comedogenic ingredient is toward the top, then it is probably present in a quantity large enough to clog pores."

4. Effectiveness

We would hope that every skin care company's goals are to create a healthy, results-driven product line free of harmful/synthetic chemicals. Unfortunately, that is not always the case. Therein lies what I choose to describe the difference between Cosmetic and Pro Level, or what should be. Most Pro Level brands represent the more results-driven products in the sense that they typically do and should use the purest form of ingredients, highest levels of the performing ingredients, free of unnecessary harmful chemicals, cruelty-free, and no artificial colorants and fragrances. But that isn't always the case. Brands that are motivated by profits only will choose to use less of the performing ingredients and more fillers, less expensive grades of ingredients, more of the harmful ingredients, as well as many synthetic colors, fragrances, and other ingredients.

Be Aware of Esoteric Marketing Terms

There are several other terms that have considerable "market value" in promoting cosmetic products to consumers, but they have very little to no meaning. Some companies actually spend money to test their products for these claims, however, most don't. Unfortunately, they are still able to get away with using these terms to sell more products.

Some of the more common terms that consumers should be aware of include:
• Dermatologist Tested
• Safe
• Hypoallergenic/Sensitivity Tested
• Fragrance Free
• Non-Comedogenic

The Make Up of a High Performance Product

There are 3 major aspects that go into creating a physically sound, healthy, results-driven product.

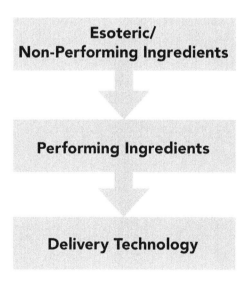

Esoteric/Non-Performing Ingredients

We want to make sure that the products have the appeal needed for a client to "want" to use it because it feels, smells, and acts well on the skin. Clients love to have the "luxury" feel at every price level. It is one of the #1 reasons why clients buy the same product over and over again.

Performing Ingredients

In order for a product to be effective, it must have the maximum potency of the key performing ingredients, yet provide a safe, positive consumer experience with no to little irritation or toxicity.

Delivery Technology

The transportation method of how to deliver the performing ingredients into the skin is key. There are some genius, new targeted delivery systems available with today's technology that can deliver ingredients with accuracy to a targeted area. We have to be able to get the corrective ingredients into the skin, for the skin to best respond to them.

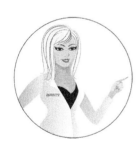

LESSON #11

"With the utilization of pharmaceutical-grade ingredients, a RESULTS-DRIVEN approach gives us a synergy between science-based and therapeutic principles of skin care, heightening the skin's ability to correct unwanted skin conditions. This significantly increases the "tools" of the Esthetician in improving the treatment of skin conditions."

Buyer Beware

Despite the reports of benefits from some skin care products, there are no requirements by the FDA to prove that the products actually live up to their claims, with the exception of sun protection products. Ultimately, it is up to the consumer to decide whether these products and their claims are valid and worth the cost, but it is our job to educate them!

Teach your clients that there are many different grades or quality of ingredients!
- **Technical Grade** – Industrial/Inexpensive/High Toxicity/Unsafe/Cheapest
- **Cosmetic Grade** – Conventional/Therapeutic in Nature/Moderately Priced
- **Food Grade** – All Natural/No Chemicals/No Preservatives/Above Average Price
- **USP (Pharmaceutical Grade)** – Pure, Healthy, Safe, Effective/Most Expensive

Simply put, higher quality means higher price. It is expensive to utilize the best-known ingredients in high concentrations.

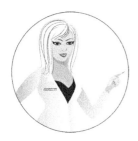

LESSON #12

"Please keep this in mind. In my experience, cheap always means cheap in skin care, however, expensive doesn't always mean good."

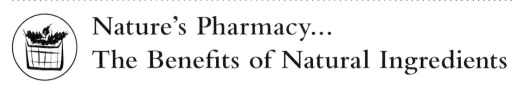

Nature's Pharmacy...
The Benefits of Natural Ingredients

A perfect marriage...natural sources along with the latest in cosmetic technology to provide a healthy way to achieve results. In the past, it always seemed that consumers had to either sacrifice healthy skin care for results, or sacrifice results to use something healthy. That is quickly changing with all old and new information about plant-based skin care. I am a huge fan of using what I call "nature's pharmacy" to create skin care products that are both safe and effective without using the harmful, synthetic ingredients found so prevalently in skin care products across all market segments.

What exactly does "natural" mean? Webster defines "natural" as "not artificial, synthetic, [or] acquired by external means," that the substance comes from a natural source, i.e. plants.

Here are some interesting facts about plant-based ingredients:
So many great skin care ingredients are derived from "natural" sources. Did you know that up to one third of all pharmaceutical drugs are also plant derived? However, many people believe that natural ingredients are not chemicals, and that they are safer. The truth is that all things are made of chemicals! There are plenty of natural things that are not safe, i.e. poison ivy contains harmful chemicals. "Natural" may mean that it is derived from nature but it is not necessarily "chemical-free", safer, or more effective. Likewise, synthetic or lab-produced ingredients do not necessarily mean that it is harmful or bad for the skin, either. I believe that we should utilize the best of both to create the best products that we can. There are effective and useful products that come from both nature and the lab.

History of Plant-Based Benefits for the Skin

Plants played a large part in Egyptian medicine and daily life well over 2,000 years ago. Plants were almost the exclusive source of cosmetics and skin care until the beginning of the 20th century. Science and the cosmetic industry have gone full circle in the discovery of benefits of plants for the skin.

Through the strides of scientific research, it is now possible to fully understand what specific plant constituents are responsible for the following skin-related benefits found in herbs, fruits and vegetables. I like to group them into two categories:

- **Skin Rejuvenation/Healing**

- **Revitalizing/Correcting**

There have been a multitude of studies that have proven that natural ingredients can have a positive physiological effect on the skin; their application in topical creams, lotions and other preparations within the traditional medicines and healing traditions of many cultures has been observed. Over the last 20 years, clinical and laboratory studies have identified the benefits of an array of natural ingredients for skin care.

There is one study that I enjoyed called "Innovations in Natural Ingredients and Their Use in Skin Care" by Fowler JF Jr, Woolery-Lloyd H, Waldorf H, Saini R. University of Louisville, Division of Dermatology, Louisville, KY 40202, USA that states, "Consequently, a number of these ingredients and compounds are today being developed, used or considered not only for anti-aging effects, but also for use in dermatologic disorders."

For example:
> Certain ingredients, such as colloidal oatmeal and aloe vera, have been identified as beneficial in the treatment of psoriasis and atopic dermatitis, respectively, due to their anti-inflammatory properties.

> For combating acne and rosacea, green tea, niacinamide and feverfew are considered efficacious.

As to hyper-pigmentation and antioxidative capabilities, red tea, licorice, green tea, alpha arbutin, soy, acai berry, turmeric and pomegranate are among those plants and compounds found to be most beneficial.

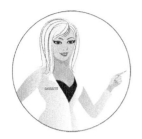

LESSON #13
"In summation…plant extracts are nature's blessings for results-driven skin care."

The Important Role of Antioxidants & Preventative Skin Care

We know now more than ever that preventative care is everything to maintain a healthy-looking and a healthy-functioning body and skin. It is critical to start practicing this as early as possible, as it is always easier to prevent than to correct damage or unwanted conditions. Carelessly treating our body becomes visibly transparent in our skin. The skin is a window to our internal health and can tell us many things about the state of our wellness and/or wellbeing.

Simply put…neglecting our health = premature aging! It is proven that antioxidants play a very important role to help us grow old healthily, and look good doing it! Antioxidants, whether from our food sources, supplements, or absorbed topically from our skin care products in addition to a healthy lifestyle, will inhibit those unwanted aging signs, which often make us feel a lack of confidence and look older than our years.

Oxidative Stress & Premature Aging

We hear so much about oxidative stress in the skin. What is oxidative stress? Oxidative stress, simply put, is the damage made to our cells through the oxidative process. Oxidation is a very normal process that inevitably happens to our bodies that usually manifests in the skin. Free oxygen radicals are created during the metabolism of normal oxygen cells, or oxidation. These free radicals are missing a simple electron and are in search of another molecule that they can combine with to become "whole." In their quest, they fire charges that damage other cells and structures around them. This, in turn, causes the collateral damage that leads to premature aging of the body and therefore, the skin. In effect, while your skin is aging as it goes through its lifetime, the free oxygen radicals are wildly running through your skin, like "Pac-Men" searching for a mate. As you can see, the more free radicals your body contains, the more damage that's likely to be done.

A Closer Look at Free Radicals

Each and every day, the human body's largest organ, the skin, is bombarded with environmental assailants resulting from exposure to smoke, pollution, and most importantly, sun exposure. Free radicals start a chain reaction under the skin's surface, therefore, the structure of our skin is damaged and its cellular structure is weakened. Free radicals also alter our DNA, which results in aging and illness.

Another factor is stress; stress produces adrenaline-related products, which not only restricts blood flow to our skin, but also generates potent, destructive free radicals. Most importantly, in the skin, free radicals trigger the release of inflammatory mediators, breaking down collagen and damaging cell barrier. In addition to this external damage, free radicals are one of the main factors contributing to the formation of cancerous cells.

What are Antioxidants & How do They Work to Fight Off Oxidative Stress?

Antioxidants have made their way front and center as important needs of the consumer. Antioxidants are **essential** to an anti-aging skin care routine. Antioxidants stand ready to repair cell damage by helping to stabilize free radicals. Antioxidants are chemicals that protect cells by neutralizing external forces (such as damage from the sun, pollution, wind, and temperature) and internal factors (for example, emotions, metabolism, and the presence of excess oxygen). Luckily, it is possible to literally boost the skin's external defenses against harmful free radicals and control environmental aging by applying antioxidants topically. These miracle cell protectors represent the front line of defense in the war against environmental aging. Countless studies have proven that antioxidants applied to the skin's surface offer protection from sun damage and stimulate collagen production.

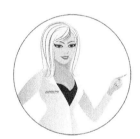

LESSON #14
"Antioxidants work from the outside in and the inside out."

The intake of antioxidants strengthens the core of our human body, and thus reflects on the outer part, which is the skin. The application of antioxidants on the outer surface of the skin can help to slow down the aging process by nurturing and "repairing" the skin. Common antioxidants in skin care are Vitamins A (Retinols), C (L-Ascorbic Acid, Magnesium Ascorbyl Phosphate), E (Tocopherol Acetate), and Beta Carotene. Let's take a closer look at some of the well-documented, results-driven antioxidants in skin care.

Vitamin C...The Antioxidant Super Hero

Vitamin C is a multi-tasker for the skin. It prevents water loss, helping to maintain the skin's barrier function, while building collagen and elastin. Furthermore, Vitamin C deactivates the unstable free radicals, preventing much of their potential damage. There is also increasing evidence that Vitamin C shields the skin from the sun's burning rays, especially when it's applied in high concentrations. Today, we have learned much about topical preparations of Vitamin C. Cosmetic chemists must carefully regulate the percentage concentration and delivery system, as these crucial variables determine the effectiveness of the product.

Other Antioxidant Ingredients

In addition to Vitamin C, there are many other powerful allies in the war against free radicals. There are many more to name that are plant/food based that are showing very promising results such as sweet potatoes, squash, pomegranates, and more. These special chemicals assist in repair of the skin, allowing us to not only prevent but to repair and correct existing damage.

When used before sun exposure, Vitamin E reduces redness and swelling of the skin, resulting in less destruction of lipids, and less sun damaged cells.

Extract of Red Tea is a powerful antioxidant. Squalene Oil is an amazing oil-soluble antioxidant. Alpha lipoic acid helps to protect the skin from sun damage by suppressing the production of the collagen-destroying enzyme, collagenase. Shea butter, rosehip oil, and sea buckthorn oil are also excellent antioxidants. It's important to know that not all antioxidants are created equal.

Additional Suggestions for Combating Oxidative Stress in the Skin

Here are several antioxidant foods, which appear the most likely to produce benefits to your skin.

- **Vitamin A or Beta Carotene.** It has been discovered that beta-carotene protects dark green, yellow and orange vegetables and fruits from sun damage, and it is thought that it plays a similar role in the human body. Carrots, squash, broccoli, sweet potatoes, tomatoes, kale, collards, cantaloupe, peaches and apricots are particularly rich sources of beta-carotene.
- **Ascorbic Acid (Vitamin C).** A water-soluble compound that fulfills an antioxidant role, among others, in living systems. Important sources include citrus fruits (like oranges, sweet lime, etc.), green peppers, broccoli, green leafy vegetables, strawberries, raw cabbage and tomatoes.
- **Vitamin E.** A principal fat-soluble antioxidant vitamin in the body. It protects cellular membranes, lipoproteins and other "oily" structures. Skin is high in unsaturated fatty acids ("oily" molecules especially susceptible to free radical damage), and can benefit from Vitamin E protection (both oral and topical). Sources include wheat germ, nuts, seeds, whole grains, green leafy vegetables, vegetable oil and fish-liver oil.
- **Flavonoids.** A diverse group of plant pigments with antioxidant properties that contain proanthocyanins and polyphenols that are good for the skin. These substances are responsible for color in many fruits, vegetables and flowers. Flavonoids provide color that attracts insects or animals, and these pigments protect plants from environmental stress. In addition to being potent antioxidants, some flavonoids have antiallergic, anticarcinogenic, antiviral and anti-inflammatory activity.

The Future of Antioxidants

As the professional skin care industry continues to explore the role of antioxidants, we are entering an exciting time to educate, protect, and deliver our clients advanced products to address a wide range of skin care concerns and slow the effects of environmental aging. Amongst the aging baby boomer generation, topical antioxidant products are increasingly in demand, both to reverse damage accumulated over years of exposure to the sun, dehydration, and environmental assailants, and to protect skin from the harmful effects of such environmental pollution.

Perhaps the most exciting development of all is the mainstream understanding and demand for antioxidants and SPF in topical skin care products. Today's average consumer is well versed and educated as to the effects of environmental damage, both from a cosmetic and a wellness perspective. As a result, antioxidant ingredients are becoming increasingly integral components of skin care, and SPF has been widely included into skin care regimens.

As we skin care professionals continue to research and develop advanced antioxidant technologies, we enter into an exciting period where Estheticians can offer the consumer the cosmetic effects of healthy skin, while providing protection against environmental damage.

Harmful Chemicals in Skin Care

I think it is important to be aware of what harmful chemicals are lurking in our industry's lotions and potions. The industry is highly unregulated and remember, there is no pre-market approval process before a product hits the market. A very minimum approval process exists, but only for color additives and ingredients classified as over-the-counter drugs.

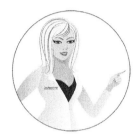

LESSON #15
"What we put on our skin gets in our skin!"

There are certain chemicals that are used in manufacturing skin care products that are known for their **proven negative effects.** Do you know that it has been scientifically proven that over ***60 percent of topically applied chemicals via cosmetics, lotions, etc. are absorbed by the skin and dispersed throughout the body by the bloodstream?*** Therefore, it is critical that we educate our clients on the avoidance of these ingredients, and recommend an alternative version for their long term safety and health of their skin and body.

Let's break it down simply. Everything is considered a chemical! Beware of the companies that claim that their products are "chemical-free"! This drives me crazy. There are good and bad chemicals as well as naturally-sourced or synthetic chemicals. What we do know is that there are thousands of chemicals in all personal care products, many of which are considered unhealthy. I personally recommend to stay away from as many synthetic chemicals as possible, however, just because an ingredient may be naturally-sourced doesn't mean it is safe, nontoxic, or won't irritate the skin.

Many of the synthetic chemicals used are what I call "triggers" or skin irritants and **are carcinogenic.** Those of you that know me know that this is a subject that I am extremely passionate about. There is MORE THAN ENOUGH EVIDENCE needed to convince me that the following chemicals should be banned based on what we know! The current studies questioning fundamental safety and the current lack of FDA testing or regulation regarding cosmetics establish a good case for avoiding these questionable ingredients all together.

In all of my studies, here are my **Top 3 Chemical Culprits** that we should avoid entirely!

#1 Chemical Culprit – Benzoyl Peroxide

Used primarily as an acne remedy, benzoyl peroxide has been linked to skin cancer for a number of years and many research journal entries state "benzoyl peroxide is a free radical-generating skin tumor promoting agent." When I recently searched the words "benzoyl peroxide and cancer" in the National Library of Medicine, I found over 102 articles from medical publications publishing the research discoveries of benzoyl peroxide and cancer. About two-thirds of the research supports linkage between benzoyl peroxide and skin cancer. I am concerned that a large percentage of our youth is still using benzoyl peroxide, and A LOT of it.

There is enough information for me to make a decision to NEVER recommend use of this ingredient, and to educate my clients on a safer alternative. I highly recommend Salicylic Acid, a naturally-derived chemical known for its antimicrobial/anti-inflammatory qualities.

#2 Chemical Culprit – Parabens

The dangers of parabens are real! The increasing concern for the safety of ingredients in cosmetics has brought some widely used cosmetic preservatives by the family name 'paraben' to center stage. Paraben preservatives are listed under multiple names, and are used to preserve the majority of cosmetics on the market today; not only to prevent the growth of bacteria and fungi, but also to promote the abnormally long shelf-life of products.

Parabens are synthetic preservatives that have been in use since the 1920s as "broad-band" preservatives (anti-bacterial and anti-fungal), which means that they work within a formula to prevent the growth of multiple possible contaminants such as bacteria, yeast, mold and fungi. They can be found in approximately 75-90 percent of cosmetics such as makeup, lotion, deodorants and shampoos.

According to *A Consumers Dictionary of Cosmetic Ingredients*, "water is the only cosmetic ingredient used more frequently than paraben preservatives". (Winter, 2005)

The US Environmental Protection Agency (EPA) in their report *Pharmaceuticals and Personal Care Products in the Environment: Agents of Subtle Change?* stated that **"the chemical preservatives called parabens – methyl, propyl, butyl and ethyl (alkyl-p-hydroxybenzoates) – displayed estrogenic activity in several tests."** This means that these chemicals mimic your body´s own hormones, and can have endocrine-disrupting action when they are rubbed into your body or washed down the drain into your drinking water. These disruptors interfere with your body´s endocrine system: your hypothalamus, your ovaries, your thyroid – virtually every system in your body. Paraben preservatives are believed to mimic the female hormone estrogen when introduced into the body. Once absorbed into the body, paraben preservatives mimic the hormone estrogen and can disrupt the body's normal hormonal balance. This artificial inflation of estrogen in the endocrine system has been linked to breast cancer in some women.

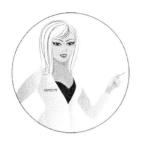

LESSON #16

"It is a known medical fact that estrogen stimulates breast cancer, and anything absorbed through the skin may be as high as 10 times the concentration of an oral dose."

Not all cosmetic companies use paraben preservatives and many are phasing out their use, now that enough concerns have been raised about their overall long term safety. Many companies are now offering "naturally-sourced" and have made their "no paraben" policy a unique selling position for their brand.

There are many safe and more natural alternatives available to preserve products. With formulas that contain certain naturally-sourced (living) ingredients and/or water as an ingredient, a more aggressive non-paraben preservative must be used to ensure the stability of the formula. The next best option is a synthetic preservative called Phenoxyethanol, which has a synthetic chemical composition inspired by a natural antibacterial/antimicrobial chemical found in the sage plant. In some formulas, a plant extract or essential oil with antimicrobial and antioxidant properties such as grapefruit seed extract or tocopherol (Vitamin E) can also be used as an effective preservative system.

The dangers of parabens may not be apparent to the point that their use is prohibited yet by the FDA, but the scientific evidence that we have to date, in my opinion, is nothing short of alarming. If you want to stay safe and use skin care products that will benefit your skin rather than harm it, it's simple… just go paraben-free.

#3 Chemical Culprit – Hydroquinone

Hydroquinone has been a go-to ingredient used for skin lightening as it reduces the production of melanin in the skin, so it is great for fading hyperpigmentation, acne marks, sun spots, melasma, and other pigmentation disruptions.

Without a doubt, hydroquinone is very effective for treating hyperpigmentation issues. However, its safety is also highly questionable. Studies have shown that hydroquinone has some carcinogenic effects when applied to skin. It is considered cytotoxic (toxic to cells) and mutagenic. Studies have also shown that long-term hydroquinone use can cause exogenous ochronosis, which is when your skin turns a bluish and black color. Hydroquinone not only inhibits melanin production to help lighten skin, but long-term use of this ingredient can actually damage skin.

Because hydroquinone decreases the melanin pigments in your skin, your skin becomes more sensitive to the sun. This increases UVA and UVB exposure, which in turn, increases the risk of getting more future hyperpigmentation, especially if you don't use a broad-spectrum, highly protective sun protection product at all times. Hydroquinone also turns toxic when exposed to sunlight, so if used, it should only be used as a spot treatment (not all over the face) at night. Aside from exogenous ochronosis and sun sensitivity, long-term hydroquinone use is also known to cause skin to get thick, leathery, and bumpy. Short-term side effects of hydroquinone include redness, irritation, and contact dermatitis. Because of these associated risks, hydroquinone has been banned in many countries in Europe and Asia.

Esthetic Equipment – My Three Faves

We have a myriad of esthetic equipment and supplies that we can use in the treatment room that are conventional, along with many new or promising modalities. Listed below are the most popular used behind the chair by Estheticians and in my opinion, the most efficacious.

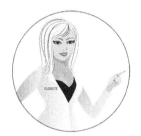

LESSON #17
"Know all of the tools in your toolbox."

Microdermabrasion

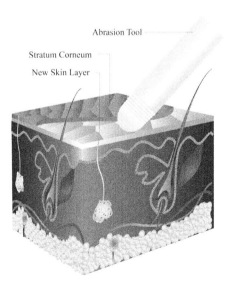

Abrasion Tool

Stratum Corneum

New Skin Layer

Microdermabrasion is one of the top requested services in spas today. It has gained steady popularity, and is now considered a "mainstay" in spas. It is a results-driven service with well-documented evidence of its efficacy for certain conditions. We can provide the next level of treatment for those clients that need corrective work, and when other services aren't enough.

It started in Europe nearly two decades ago, and has been performed in the United States since 1993. It is the most natural way to evenly and safely exfoliate the skin without chemicals within our scope of practice.

What is Microdermabrasion?
Microdermabrasion is a mechanical exfoliation technique that works from the outside in, as it buffs and polishes the surface of the skin. Microdermabrasion removes approximately 1-2 microns of depth of skin. Exfoliation is the process of removing these dead skin cells and debris, and improving the superficial texture of the skin. By taking off these dead cells the skin has a smoother, healthier appearance. It also works from the inside out as it can stimulate collagen to create a toned, tightened effect to the skin through the vacuum "massaging" of the skin.

What conditions improve with Microdermabrasion
- Non-inflamed acne
- Acne scars
- Age spots
- Discoloration
- Fine lines & wrinkles
- Sun damaged skin
- Uneven, rough skin texture
- Tightening and toning effect

Clients with the following conditions should avoid Microdermabrasion
- Active herpes lesions
- Active pustular acne
- Rosacea
- Open sores or lesions
- Dermatitis
- Psoriasis
- People using Accutane within the last 12 months
- Eczema

The best results come from understanding that microdermabrasion has a cumulative result. Although clients will see and feel a difference in the skin following just one treatment, the real results come with multiple sessions at monthly intervals or more frequently if needed, yielding long-term results.

Chemical Peels

Chemical peels have long been a favorite amongst most Estheticians. There are many variables to peel solutions on the market. Please remember that all peel solutions cannot be treated equally. Each manufacture's solutions may have different percentages (strength), different pH levels, treatment times, treatment protocols, some are neutralized and some are not, and so on. Be sure to follow each manufacturer's directions accordingly to eliminate the potential for problems.

How do Chemical Peels work? Instantly, when applied to the face or another part of the body, the peel solution works by removing the outer layers of skin so that a new, smooth layer of skin is revealed. Cumulatively, these peels have longer lasting effects such as texture improvement, tightening, more even pigmentation/tone, and overall healthier appearance.

Topically, AHA (glycolic/lactic) acids dissolve desmosomes, the protein bridges that hold dead skin cells together, resulting in a fresher, more youthful appearance. Topically, BHA (salicylic) works by creating desquamation (shedding) as a means of exfoliation. From the inside out, the action of the chemicals can stimulate the production of fibroblasts, which in turn creates collagen, essential components of healthy, toned, youthful skin.

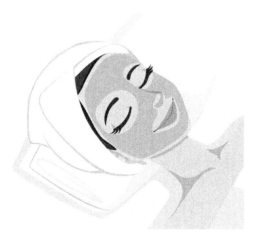

In general, clients with fair skin and light hair are the best chemical peel candidates. However, clients with other skin pigmentation and hair color can achieve good results as well. Ideal candidates for the chemical peel procedure are individuals who are unhappy with the appearance of their skin, and have realistic expectations of their procedure.

What conditions improve with Chemical Peels
- Reduces fine lines and wrinkles
- Improves disoloration
- Treats certain types of acne
- Improves the texture of the skin
- Improves sun damage

Clients with the following conditions should avoid Chemical Peels
- Active herpes lesions
- Active pustular acne
- Rosacea
- Open sores or lesions
- Dermatitis
- Psoriasis
- People using Accutane within the last 12 months
- Eczema
- Any known allergies to the source of the solution
- Recent sun exposure

Ultrasound

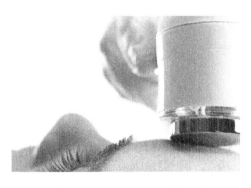

What is an **Ultrasound Facial?** This high-tech facial uses a specialized ultrasonic/ultrasound modality that emits waveforms into the skin. Ultrasonic treatments benefit a variety of skin types, and can improve many common skin conditions. Ultrasound works in a myriad of ways to promote healthy skin. These waveforms stimulate body cells; the micro massage it produces expands the space in which the cells exist, causing movement of cytoplasm, the rotation of mitochondria, and the vibration of the cell nucleus. It stimulates and expands the cell's membrane. It improves local blood and lymph circulation, and increases the absorption quality of the skin through thermal warming caused by these waveforms. In turn, it enhances product delivery, allowing us to target specific conditions with the infusion of the appropriate serum used along with ultrasound in treatment.

Ultrasonic Facial has 4 distinct functions to improve the metabolism and regeneration of the skin cells.

1) Warming and Heating Function

The heat is produced by vigorous friction of the modules in speed vibration. To healthy cells, heat supplies energy and speeds metabolism. The warming and heating action is one of the most important therapeutic factors of ultrasound. It is a type of internal heat, an increase of about 79-80%; this heat is carried away by the blood circulation and is not perceived by the client. This warming action can change the blood circulation and helps to reduce inflammation. It is also of great benefit to reduce swelling, encourage the healing process, and to reduce puffiness. It produces a relaxing and comforting effect on the client.

2) Mechanical Function

Cavitation occurs when the ultrasonic waves are surging through the skin. Cavitation means "bubbles". The mechanical results help to clean pores, stimulate the skin, increase cell turnover, can create new collagen formation, and produce a mild exfoliation on the surface of the skin.

3) Vibratory Function

This high-speed vibration (machinery affect) action on the tissue is just like massage. It stimulates the release of toxins and waste products out of the cells, and transfers them into the lymphatic system. Another byproduct of ultrasonic therapy is increased blood supply, which promotes healing.

4) Chemical/Infusion Function

Small doses of ultrasound treatments can promote the synthesis of protein inside the cells, help to regenerate wounded tissues, and promote the synthesis of fiber cells in the body. In the process of anabolism and catabolism, the induced product is being absorbed and utilized by the cells. The accelerated metabolism of the cells changes the pH level of the skin to a more alkaline state, and facilitates the absorption of the induced product.

What conditions improve with Ultrasound

- Exfoliates dead skin cells for clear and radiant skin
- Loosens and removes oil, dirt and sebum from the pores and hair follicles, resulting in less blackheads and breakouts
- Gently stimulates skin to encourage collagen production
- With a series of treatments, fine lines and wrinkles are less noticeable; skin color, tone and texture becomes more even and uniform
- Stimulates blood flow and lymphatic drainage through the combination of ultrasound and electrical therapy; nourishes the skin and gives it a youthful rosy glow
- Facilitates hydration and plumps the skin, thereby filling out fine lines and wrinkles
- Helps skin care products do their job by penetrating deeper into the skin (this is especially true for anti-aging and antioxidant serums)

Clients with the following conditions should avoid Ultrasonic Facials

This modality is safe for most people. The sonic waves emitted by the ultrasound machine aren't harmful to your health. However, if you have an autoimmune disorder, a diagnosed heart disorder or cancer, implants or metal devices, it's best to skip the ultrasonic treatment.

- Never use on irritated skin
- Do not use on pregnant women
- Always use ultrasonic electrodes with sufficient media (herbal spray or serum on the skin)

THE TREATMENT BEGINS...

"It is so important that we meet the reasonable expectations of our clients' needs. Creating a treatment plan that yields results is critical."

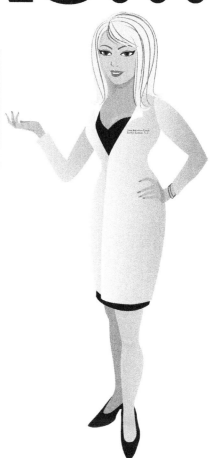

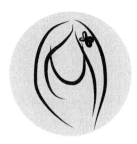

How to Conduct an Effective Skin Analysis

Now that we've refreshed our memories about the skin and how it functions, and what tools that we have to work with, we can now "prescribe" a more accurate approach to the care of the skin. The next step is performing an effective consultation and skin analysis. Why is the consultation and the skin analysis the most important part of the process? It allows us to bond or "cement" the relationship with our clients, and provides the best opportunity for educating the client.

Here are a couple of things I want you to try, to improve your consultations. After escorting the client to the room, ask them to change into the wrap provided, and sit on the facial table to wait for you. Don't let them get tucked in quite yet. We want their full attention as we go through questions with them. Once they get "tucked in" between the linens, we tend to lose much of their attention.

When you re-enter the treatment room, go over the skin care questionnaire. For return clients, be sure that nothing has changed since their last visit, such as new medications, pregnancy, new products, etc. Before you ask them to lie down and get tucked in to perform the skin analysis, ask them the following questions.
- What do you currently like about your skin?
- Are you having any problems with your skin?
- What would you like to see improved?
- What would you change if you could?

Then, once you listen carefully to both the physical challenges facing your client's skin and to her feelings related to those challenges, be sure to write all of the information down on her paperwork/client profile.

Next, tuck the client in and make sure that she is comfortable. Now is when you will pre-cleanse the skin and perform the skin analysis. It is VERY important that as we look at our client's skin, we validate the concerns that they shared, and educate them on what we see. **This is a perfect time to create the treatment plan!** The best thing to do is to deflect that information back to them. It may sounds something like this, "I see the fine lines on your upper lip that concern you. I am also seeing a bit of sun damage here. Are you interested in hearing about what services and products I recommend to improve that?" We know that they will be interested because they have already shared their concerns about most of it.

Next, describe in detail the best treatment plan (services and product) for them, based on treating their most predominant condition first. I would suggest that you try to get a commitment of at least three visits. Simply ask them if they are ready to get started on that today! Then, plan what will take place with each visit. Clients love to know that you have a plan, and that it's customized to their needs!

The 3–3's...My Basic Principles for Creating Results-Oriented Treatment Plans

Now, let's apply what we know about the client's needs and wants. Throughout my career, I never thought of myself as an Esthetician that provides that "feel good" facial. As you will experience throughout reading this book, I take what we do seriously, and my approach has been and still is a more clinical approach to the treatment of skin. Results are everything! So before we can achieve results, we must first have a plan. Remember that what we do is two-fold; results come from both 1) services that we offer and 2) the products that we recommend for home care. We need to understand everything from cosmetic chemistry, ingredients and formulas, and what each can do to benefit the skin, as well as to understand the dynamics and benefits of esthetic equipment, i.e. microdermabrasion, high frequency, steamers, etc. Once we really know all of the "tools in our tool box", we can then create a Treatment Plan for our clients that yield results.

Creating a Treatment Plan for your clients does several things:

- A client "buys in" to the concept that multiple services are recommended and needed, to achieve goals and experience long lasting results. Oftentimes, you can offer incentives for them to pre-book a series this way, i.e. "buy 5, receive the 6th one free", etc. This also builds your book of business quickly.

- Clients like to know that you have customized a plan for them, and they are most likely going to follow a plan.

- A client tends to invest more often in your home care regimen recommendations, when it is presented as part of the plan.

When it comes to the successful treatment of skin, we must ascertain many things about each individual client's skin, before we can accurately determine the best plan/approach to reach their goals. Most of us, however, struggle with the consultation process. I have developed a very simple, successful approach. I call it the 3-3's.

The **3-3**'s to Your Skin Analysis

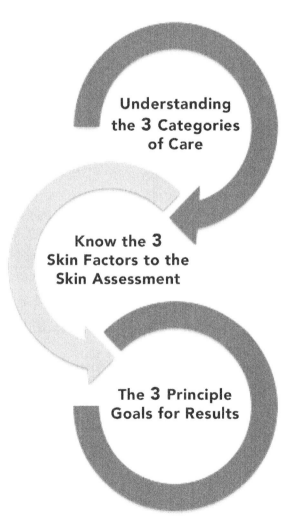

Understanding the 3 Categories of Care

Know the 3 Skin Factors to the Skin Assessment

The 3 Principle Goals for Results

The **3** Categories of Care

Based on the skin assessment, there are 3 Categories of Care that we can offer. It is helpful to make a determination as to what category your clients fall into, how progressive you may need to be, how frequent they visit you to meet the goal, etc.

Preventative Care

This is typically your younger, healthier skin type with very little to no unwanted conditions. Perhaps they are a bit more aware of the fact that taking care of their skin early counts. It may also be a client that is maturing and wants to maintain the current health and appearance of their skin. Creating a treatment plan for this client would be geared more towards keeping the skin in great shape. Regular facials, exfoliation services (such as microdermabrasion, enzyme exfoliants, scrubs and peels) are all great recommendations. Home care would be focusing on hydrators, antioxidants and sunscreens.

Corrective Care

This is our more typical client. This is our largest demographic of client type. The average age group of this type is anywhere from age 14 to 65. This is the client who is coming in to seek your professional advice because he/she has present unwanted conditions they want to see improved. They are generally prepared and ready to make a commitment to you. These are the perfect clients to create that long-term skin wellness plan for. Most often we may need to recommend the more progressive types of services, how frequently they receive them, and how many they need, for this type of client.

Maintenance Care

Once we reach a client's skin care goals, we need to educate them on the need for maintenance. Nothing we can do for their skin lasts forever. We can modify, persuade, and coax the skin into doing many things with our products and services, but unless there is a maintenance plan in place, the results may fade in time. The maintenance care is also both in services and products.

The 3 Skin Factors to the Skin Assessment

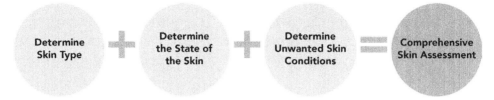

1. Determine the **Skin Type**. Choose One:
   a. Normal
   b. Water Dry (Dehydrated)
   c. Oil Dry (Lacking Oil)
   d. Oily
   e. Combination

Our goal is to balance the oil and water in the skin. This helps us to determine if we are going to be utilizing water or oil, or combination types of base products for their service and for home care recommendations.

2. Determine the **State of the Skin** (Inflamed or Non-Inflamed). Choose One:
   a. Inflamed/Erythema/Warm to Touch/Red
   b. Non-Inflamed/Sluggish/Congested/Dull in Color
   c. Combination

The goal is to normalize the state of the skin. This helps us to determine whether we are going to stimulate or sedate (or both) the skin throughout the service and home care recommendations.

3. Determine what **Skin Conditions** are present. Choose All That Apply:
   a. Acne
   b. Milia
   c. Hyperpigmentation
   d. Fine Lines/Wrinkles
   e. Sun Damage
   f. Laxity (Sagging)
   g. Rosacea

The goal is to correct unwanted conditions. I like to recommend that you begin with the most prominent skin condition first. This helps us to determine the corrective ingredient(s) we are going to be utilizing for their service and home care recommendations.

The **3** Principle Goals for Results

I practice by **3 Principles/Goals** to achieve healthy skin. It's what I call the **"BNC"** for corrective skin care – **Balance, Normalize, Correct**.
This applies to both professional services and home care.

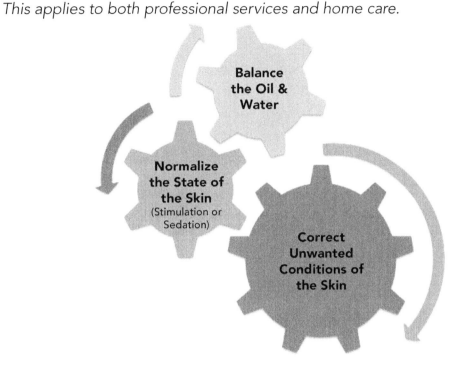

Balance – The Hydrolipidic Film (Oil/Water Content in the Skin)

It all starts here! If the skin is out of balance, it does not function properly. When it doesn't function properly, it starts to show unhealthy signs. The skin functions at its optimum when there is balance of both oil and water in the skin. Please keep in mind that there is a big difference between oil dry and water dry. They can have very similar appearances, but we would treat and recommend products differently for each type. EVERYONE is water dry! We know that that the skin cannot "water" itself to adequate levels needed to have balance. Based on our client's skin type, if the skin is lacking water we need to hydrate it, if the skin is lacking oil we need to supplement it with oil. If the skin is lacking both water and oil, give it both! Regardless, it is imperative that the skin remains balanced with the adequate amount of both. This helps you to determine what products (whether oil-based or water-based, or both) are needed.

Normalize the State of the Skin (Inflamed or Non-Inflamed)

It is critical that the skin remains in a balanced, non-inflamed state. Inflammation can be directly related to premature aging and many other unwanted skin disorders and diseases. The goal would be to sedate and calm this skin state. On the other hand, a dull, lifeless appearance to the skin may be improved through stimulation. We can normalize the state of the skin through stimulation and sedation methods with both equipment and products. In order to do that, we must first determine if the skin is inflamed or non-inflamed. They usually are distinctly different, although, you may sometimes see a combination of both.

Inflamed Skin Characteristics
- Redness (Erythema)
- Swelling (Edema)
- Feels Warm to Touch
- Soreness
- Pustular Activity

*If the skin is inflamed, recommend **sedative** services and products to calm and soothe.*

Non-Inflamed Skin Characteristics
- Sluggishness
- Sallow Color
- Congestion
- Rough Texture
- Skin Thickness

*If the skin is non-inflamed, recommend **stimulating** services and products.*

Correct Unwanted Conditions of the Skin

We can successfully correct unwanted conditions with the proper services and products. Estheticians can directly control esthetic conditions on the surface of the skin and indirectly control them below the surface. Choose the "Condition Specific" products that will address these conditions for the client's home care regimen.

- Congestion (Milia, Comedones, Keratinized Skin)
- Acne (Inflamed/Non-Inflamed)
- Enlarged Pores
- Laxity (Sagging)
- Pigmentary Problems (Melasma, Chloasma, Post-Inflammatory Pigmentation from Lesions)
- Oxidative Stress (Caused by Environmental Damage, Diet, Lifestyle, Sun Exposure, Illness, Medications)
- Fine Lines/Wrinkles
- Rough Texture

Example: If a client has water dry skin, with inflammation, along with comedones, the treatment plan/goal would look like this: You would prominently use/recommend water-based (balance), anti-inflammatory (sedate to normalize), and emulsifying (to correct conditions) treatments and products.

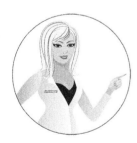

LESSON #18

"Based on the outcome of the skin assessment, create your customized BNC treatment plan for that client."

Ultimate Goals for Healthy Skin... The "Mattress" Theory

I have been teaching the "mattress" theory for years. Envision the skin simply broken down into two pieces like that of a mattress and a fitted sheet.

- The goal with the mattress (Dermis) would be to create a firm, plump, pliable, integral foundation. This is accomplished through stimulation of collagen, increased hydration, and increased oxygen and blood flow.
- The goal with the fitted sheet (Epidermis) would be to keep it clean, wrinkle-free, free of discoloration, tight fitting, and soft. This is accomplished through exfoliation, brightening, increased cellular proliferation, increased hydration, and lubrication.

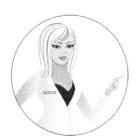

LESSON #19

"If you follow my simple BNC Formula, you will begin to see positive changes in your client's skin."

Identifying the Most Common Skin Conditions & Their Anecdotes

We as Estheticians can directly influence certain conditions on the surface of the skin, and indirectly influence them from the inside out. Properly recognizing the common skin conditions below can assist you in performing a more accurate skin assessment, and in turn, assist in determining the appropriate treatment plan (procedure protocol and home care products) to minimize their appearance and achieve optimum results.

Skin Condition	My #1 Home Care Anecdote
Large Pores Pores, or follicular openings, are seen in a variety of shapes and sizes. The size or diameter of a pore is related to the amount of sebum (oil) production, hereditary factors and the lack of elasticity in the skin.	Salicylic Acid to keep the follicles clean. This in itself can reduce the appearance of larger pores due to evacuation of the entire filament within the pore.

Skin Condition	My #1 Home Care Anecdote
Dehydration This is also known as TEWL (Transepidermal Water Loss). Dehydration is the most common esthetic skin condition. The skin takes on a tissue-like appearance. This can be caused by lack of moisture (water) excreted by the eccrine gland, or environmentally by sun damage, heat, improper cleansing and care, excessive use of retinoic acids, AHAs, BHAs or other low pH topicals.	Hyaluronic Acid to rehydrate the skin and allow it to function adequately. We know that the skin cannot produce and retain the level of water that it needs on its own. When the skin is hydrated, it looks, feels, and functions better. When the skin is dehydrated it is also common to see many other unwanted skin conditions arise such as fine lines, itchiness, increased sensitivity levels and more.
Milia Milia is a sebaceous (oil) gland condition. These small, keratinized cysts get lodged within the epidermis. They can be found most anywhere, but usually more prominent under the eyes and on the external areas of the face. They can be sometimes be removed carefully by creating an opening in the skin with a lancet and a comedone extractor. For larger ones or deeply embedded ones, the client may need to seek a Dermatologist to remove them.	I have had great success using Salicylic Acid as a spot treatment, as it helps to proliferate to the surface quicker, and help to dry and shrink the size of the milia. Once they are more surfaced, I recommend 100% Squalane Oil to emulsify and soften the sebum. This can be dabbed directly on the milia at night.

Skin Condition	My #1 Home Care Anecdote
Comedones/Blackheads There are both open comedones and closed comedones. These are recognizable by a hardened, darkened, sometimes-raised filament that is congested and made up of a mixture of dead skin cells, sebum (oil), environmental debris, and water. The filament on the surface turns darker due to oxidation with the air. These may be successfully removed by several methods. Softening the filament with moist heat and extraction softeners before extraction, works extremely well to correct this condition.	I love Salicylic Acid for both open and closed comedones. I often refer to Sal Acid as "drano for the pores". It is an ideal tool to produce the antimicrobial effect that we need to control bacterial growth in the pores, as well as it acts as an excellent anti-inflammatory agent to relieve any inflammation that may be present.
Distended Capillaries/ Telangiectasia These are vascular structures found close to the surface of the skin, or there had been a dilation of the capillary structure making the capillary appear broken. Distended capillaries are created by several factors. Genetics play a big role in the makeup of our capillary structure but can be worsened by environmental factors. Sun damage can cause irreversible capillary distention, resulting in a ruddy-like complexion. Stimulants in the body such as caffeine, tobacco smoke, drugs, and alcohol can increase capillary distention. Telangiectasia is a term used for a permanent area of distended or damaged capillaries.	The best remedy for effecting these types of vascular conditions is to use topical "sedatives" to calm and create the vasoconstrictive action needed to relieve the skin of the inflammation and heat associated with these conditions. My favorite naturally-sourced sedative for the skin is Chyrannthelum Indicum derived from the Daisy plant as well as colloidal ingredients, such as magnesium, copper and colbalt. Keep in mind that we can improve the appearance of these conditions. We cannot expect to "repair" vascular damage but we can help to manage the appearance the conditions associated with it.

What are common skin conditions you encounter when you perform your skin analysis?

_____
_____
_____
_____
_____
_____
_____
_____
_____
_____

How have you treated these skin conditions in the past?

_____
_____
_____
_____
_____
_____
_____
_____
_____
_____

What home care products will you now recommend?

_____
_____
_____
_____
_____
_____
_____
_____
_____
_____

An Important Note About Cold Sores Detected During Skin Assessment

The Herpes Virus is also known as herpes simplex virus 1 (HSV1). It is typically the cause of cold sores around the mouth. They are contagious and are usually spread from skin-to skin contact with an infected person through small breaks in the skin or mucous membrane. The HSV1 virus is more likely to be spread through things like implements, utensils, and towels from a person who has an active lesion. Shingles is also a HSV.

Clients that have an active Herpes breakout/ condition are contraindicated to ALL Services until completely healed. Utensils, towels, water, glasses, sheets and other commonly used items can spread the virus when blisters are pre-existing.

COMMON HEALTH RELATED ISSUES **THAT EFFECT THE SKIN**

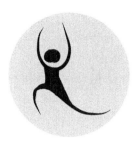

Skin Conditions Associated with Health Issues

Each time you perform a treatment on a client that may have health challenges, please be aware of any medications that the client is currently taking. We need to understand what side effects could occur on the skin resulting from the medications. Medications can affect or interfere in some way with esthetics treatments that you perform or products that you provide. I suggest that you get yourself a copy of the Physician's Desk Reference (PDR), so that you can quickly determine if there are any contraindications. Listed below are some of the most common health challenged conditions that we see with our clients.

A Note About Sensitive Skin

According to Dermatologist Dr. Leslie Baumann, there are **four types of sensitive skin:** *acne*, *rosacea*, *burning* and *stinging*, and *dermatitis*. Baumann claims that these skin types all have one characteristic in common: INFLAMMATION. Inflammation of the skin should be avoided at all times if possible. There is a direct correlation to premature aging and other skin disorders due to chronic inflammation.

1. ACNE
Can be an inflammatory skin condition that results in superficial skin lesions. These breakouts may or may not become infected with the Propionibacterium acnes (P. acnes) bacteria that live within the hair follicles. The function of sebum, which contains lactic acid and fatty acids, is to lubricate the skin. Both acids inhibit the growth of pathogenic bacteria, which are always anxious to thrive.

When sebum is unable to flow and gets trapped by either clogged pores or glands that have been damaged, it breaks or damages some of the cells lining the sebum tracts, and inflammation occurs.

2. ROSACEA

A chronic, but treatable, inflammatory skin condition that occurs in various grades. The face, neck, and chest can be marked by flushing, slight breakouts, heat, and distended capillaries. The cause of rosacea is not completely known, but theories range from bacteria, genetic causes, side effects of sun exposure, and vascular issues.

3. CHRONIC BURNING/STINGING

The cause is somewhat unknown. Anecdotal science shows that soothing, cooling compresses or products can help reduce the sensation of burning and stinging. Typically, this is thought to be brought on by allergens of some sort.

Allergens: When an individual is allergic to an ingredient, their immune system makes antibodies against the ingredient to which they are allergic, thus causing a reaction on the skin. The most common culprits in skin care are mostly fragrance, preservatives, colors, or additional harsh, and other synthetic chemicals.

Irritants: This is when a substance is irritating to the skin, but an individual is not allergic to it. For example, if you put Vitamin C on your skin you could be irritated by it, but it doesn't mean you are allergic to it.

4. DERMATITIS

Contact Dermatitis. A very common problem manifesting on the hands as red, dry, scaly, and cracked skin.

Atopic Dermatitis. Considered a more severe condition, normally associated with inflammation.

How to Balance, Normalize and Correct for Results

STRESS

How we are coping on the inside may be affecting how we look on the outside. Studies link factors such as stress, depression, and anxiety to an increase in skin problems.

Stress can manifest in the skin primarily by making the skin more sensitive and more reactive.

Stress also is a known to trigger or worsen fever blisters, "cold sores," psoriasis, seborrheic dermatitis, and has even been shown to impair skin barrier function and dehydrate the skin.

Skin Conditions Associated With This Health Issue
Hives, Irritation, Acne Breakouts, Dilated Capillaries, Warmth, Telangiesctasia, Rosacea.

Recommended Services – Calming Facials. Microdermabrasion and peels are not advised if any reactive or contraindicated skin conditions are present. Calming services can be just what the client needs to unwind and de-stress.

BNC Goals:		
Balance:		Water & Oil
Normalize:		Sedate
Correct:		Calming Serums, Antioxidants, Hydrators

DIABETES

Diabetes is a chronic health condition where the body is unable to produce enough insulin and properly break down sugar (glucose) in the blood.

Skin Conditions Associated With This Health Issue

Some individuals who have type 2 diabetes have patches of dark, velvety skin. High blood sugar levels prevent white blood cells from functioning normally. When these cells do not function properly, wounds take much longer to heal and become infected more frequently.

Thickening of the Skin: This can be localized. Common underlying pathogenesis involves biochemical alterations in dermal collagen and mucopolysaccharides.

Recommended Services – Calming services designed for sensitive skin. While clients with diabetes may have poor wound healing abilities, this should not be a factor in an enzyme exfoliation, microdermabrasion, or mild peel. No specific precautions need to be taken for these procedures, since they are limited to the epidermis – the most superficial layer of the skin. Light microdermabrasion performed by an experienced Esthetician can eliminate rough, dry patches seen with this condition.

BNC Goals:	Balance:	Water & Oil
	Normalize:	Sedate
	Correct:	Calming Serums, Hydrators, Gentle Exfoliants

HYPERTENSION (High Blood Pressure)

High blood pressure (HBP) or hypertension means high pressure (tension) in the arteries. Arteries are vessels that carry blood from the pumping heart to all the tissues and organs of the body.

Skin Conditions Associated With This Health Issue
While high blood pressure does not cause many side effects that would affect a facial treatment, the medications taken for hypertension can have side effects such as vascular dilation (redness), dizziness, fatigue, cold hands and feet, skin rash, and may require adjustments to the spa treatment.

Recommended Services – Most Facials will be ok. Microderm-abrasion and peels are not advised if any reactive or contraindi-cated skin conditions are present. Redness might occur with any service and be prolonged after the services.

BNC Goals:	Balance:	Water & Oil
	Normalize:	Sedate
	Correct:	Calming Serums, Hydrators

MENOPAUSE

Menopause is the time in a woman's life when the function of the ovaries ceases.

Skin Conditions Associated With This Health Issue

Changes in skin texture and hydration levels may develop along with worsening of acne in those affected by this condition. The loss of estrogen during menopause makes the skin, dry, thin, experience laxity, and transparency.
Some Sensitivities, Dull Complexion, Acne, Pigmentation Abnormalities.

Recommended Services – All Facials would be ok. Microderm-abrasion and peels are not advised if any reactive, thin, or contra-indicated skin conditions are present; otherwise they are good.

BNC Goals:	Balance:	Water & Oil
	Normalize:	Stimulate or Sedate
	Correct:	Calming Serums, Hydrators

CONTACT DERMATITIS

Dermatitis is an inflammation of the skin of which there are two types:

1. **Allergic Contact Dermatitis** often results from an immune response within 24-48 hours of contact with the causing agent. It typically results from exposure to certain plants, chemical additives, fragrances, preservatives and emulsifiers in skin care products, and some medications.
2. **Irritant Contact Dermatitis** results from coming in contact with a substance that is directly damaging and irritating to your skin. No allergy is required, and it will occur on the first exposure. The longer the substance remains on the skin, the more severe the reaction.

Skin Conditions Associated With This Health Issue
Determining the differences between allergic contact dermatitis and irritant contact dermatitis can be difficult.
- A red rash is the usual reaction. It appears immediately in irritant contact dermatitis, but in allergic contact dermatitis, the rash does not appear for one to two days after the exposure.
- Skin may develop small fluid filled structures (vesicles) that can cause weeping, a characteristic of these sorts of eruptions.

Recommended Services – No peels or microdermabrasion should be performed on a client with these symptoms. Just Hydrating, Calming, Soothing Facials with a mild exfoliating step.

BNC Goals:	Balance:	Water & Oil
	Normalize:	Sedate
	Correct:	Calming Serums, Hydrators

Common Skin Conditions & Suggested Ingredients That Correct Them

CONDITION: **ERYTHEMA** (Inflammation, Swelling)
GOAL: Diffuse Redness/Inflammation, Calm

Ingredients To Correct:

Salix Alba (Willow) Bark Extract – Contains a compound called salicin, which is a natural anti-inflammatory and analgesic.

Chamomile – A renowned botanical that is famous for its anti-irritant and anti-redness.

Butyrospermum Parkii (Shea Butter) – Shea butter is an anti-inflammatory, anti-irritant, highly emollient, and is high in Vitamin E.

Ginkgo Biloba Leaf Extract – Antioxidant and anti-inflammatory; supports collagen synthesis.

Vitamin E – Antioxidant protects from oxidative stress, anti-inflammatory.

Zinc Oxide – Natural zinc oxide is the perfect calming ingredient.

CONDITION: **DEHYDRATION** (Rough Texture)
GOAL: Hydrate

Ingredients To Correct:

Allantoin (found in the leaves of the Comfrey Plant) – Has healing and soothing benefits, and provides maximum hydration.

Leucine (L) derived from Soybeans – A protein source containing phospholipids; emulsifier, emollient, moisturizing.

Olea Europaea Squalane (Olive Oil) – Contains unsaturated fatty acids, polyphenols, Vitamin E, tocopherols and squalane that together help soften and moisturize.

Rosa Canina (Rose Hip) Fruit Oil – Unique in that it contains retinol, while most plants do not. High levels of Vitamin C, minerals, and essential fatty acids make it a perfect oil for moisturizing and soothing dry, fragile, or compromised skin.

Hyaluronic Acid (HA) – Holds water in the skin to plump and hydrate.

CONDITION: **STINGING, BURNING**
GOAL: Soothe, Calm

Ingredients To Correct:

Menthol – Cooling, refreshing ingredient that works its magic as an analgesic, anti-irritant, anti-itch and antimicrobial, protecting the skin while easing discomfort.

Panthenol (D) – Naturally moisturizing and protecting power hitter improves hydration while reducing itching and inflammation of the skin.

Colloidals – Strong anti-inflammatory qualities.

Azulene – Is thought to assist in calming a wide variety of skin irritations and conditions because of its soothing properties, anti-inflammatory effects and antibacterial properties.

Chrysanthellum Indicum – This extract has a well-documented effect on vascular wall permeability and increase of the mechanical resistance of capillaries.

Please Note: *Based on the possible skin conditions caused by health challenges and or the medications taken to control the situation, keep the professional and home care regimen simple. It is the responsibility of the Esthetician/skin care specialist to seek out skin care products that are formulated specifically for health challenged skin; i.e. free of unnecessary harmful chemicals, low pH, abrasive, heat inducing, etc.*

Tips on Working with Oncology Clients

In working with oncology clients undergoing cancer treatments, the skin can be compromised and pose challenges for Estheticians such as hyper-dehydration, increased sensitivity levels, blood clot risks, influencing lymph nodes, thinned skin, and loss of elasticity. Estheticians must know their products and services in depth and have the ability to modify their skin care product applications, tools, techniques, and equipment in order to adapt for the conditions associated with side effects of the cancer treatments and how they effect the skin.

In addressing each client's own specific conditions, Estheticians start by establishing whether they are working with a client in active treatment, a recent finish and now in recovery, or someone in long-term treatment. This helps us to determine the best treatment course, length, frequency, tolerability and the like. I make strong recommendations that clients seeking treatment should be seeking their physician's approval before moving forward with any service and/or home care regimen.

In working with clients still in active cancer treatment or recent recovery, the skin is usually extremely dry and dehydrated, inflamed and irritated, fragile, sun sensitive, and can be very reactive. In this situation, treat the most predominant condition, *sensitivity*, first. Focus on hydrating, soothing, calming and gentle services, with a very simple home care regimen.

Be sure to stay away from low pH-based products, irritants such as artificial fragrances and colorants, detergent-based ingredients such as ammonium lauryl sulphate or phosphates, and acid-based formulas that strip the lipids and proteins of the stratum corneum. Focus on products and services that moisturize with ingredients such as emollients, humectants, and occlusive ointments.

In addition, avoid excessive heat, steam, hot towels, too progressive or too irritating services. Avoid harsh or physical exfoliants, retinol-based products, chemical peels, alcohols, astringents, or anything that could dry the skin. I advise that no extractions be performed, because of the potential for excessive bleeding, potential bruising, unnecessary inflammation, and the very serious risk of cross-contamination or infection.

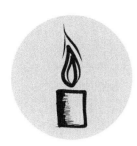

Inflammation & Aging...
The Perfect Storm

It has been well proven that chronic inflammation is linked to some of the most feared illnesses, as well as aging. Importantly, the cellular links between inflammation, disease, cancer and aging have recently been established and recognized.

Skin concerns are separated into two basic categories:
- Acute (short term)
- Chronic (long term)

Three major irritants that effect the skin barrier and can cause inflammation:
- Environmental (smoking, allergens, UV rays and pollution)
- Hormonal (stress and acne)
- Physical (harsh products, medical/cosmetic procedures)

Why does inflammation occur? Acute inflammation is triggered to repair the damaged skin barrier by repurposing the injured skin. The body does not know when to stop "fixing" itself and continues to produce pro-inflammatory molecules to ensure the problem is corrected. This type of temporary inflammation is not as harmful to the skin, whereas, chronic or long-term inflammation can wreak havoc. Chronic inflammation results in breakdown of collagen, elastin, increase in oil production, and an increase in free radicals. The good news is that certain topical skin care products can prevent acute inflammation from becoming chronic.

Inflammation & Skin Disease

In the last decade, the scientific community has determined that inflammation and disease can go hand in hand. The incidence of skin cancer has reached epidemic proportions. The most common procedures still performed today by dermatologists relate to skin cancer therapy. These surgical procedures treating skin cancer rose by 12% to include more than 1.7 million, despite massive public education on the relationship of sunlight to skin cancer. This trend is increasing, despite the introduction of sunscreens in the 1980s.

Sun Exposure & Inflammation

It has been documented that even the smallest doses of UV light induce chronic inflammation and tissue damage. Repeated chronic irritation of the skin due to any cause has been proven to produce long-term inflammation. Important: Acute inflammation followed by rapid complete repair of the skin barrier does not appear to induce skin damage, therefore, not resulting in visible skin aging.

Inflammation can Wreak Havoc on How Your Skin Looks as You Age

Chronic inflammation can accelerate your skin's aging process. Inflammation is an essential part of the body's healing process. It occurs at the cellular level when the immune system tries to fight off disease-causing germs and repair injured tissue. However, long-term inflammation can be dangerous. The correlation of chronic inflammation and skin aging and cancer was suggested years ago. It is now clear that detrimental, chronic inflammation can be prevented and reversed by a healthy diet, oral supplements, *as well as the application of topical skin care products and services.* In cases of chronic inflammation, the immune system starts perceiving the body's tissues as foreign and thereby, posing a threat. As a result, it can produce dynamics to destroy the tissue while trying to rebuild it. This can lead to a number of other unwanted skin conditions, such as dermatitis, psoriasis, eczema and acne.

Aging of the Skin

In their mid-twenties, human beings reach the peak of their growth and development. Age is marked by biological changes. The speed and degree to which an individual will age is a complex and cumulative combination of genetics, environment and lifestyle.

There are two theories as to why we age. One is the pre-programmed theory, which suggest we all have a biological clock that keeps ticking over a lifetime following a predetermined genetic timetable. The second one is environmental exposure to the skin that causes cumulative and progressive damage.

The aging process begins the minute we are born. We **absolutely** can preserve our skin health through comprehensive maintenance or care. Just like all other organs, the skin also slows down as we age. Therefore, we need to supplement the skin just as we do for the rest of our bodies.

Two Types of Aging
- Intrinsic Aging
- Influenced Aging

Intrinsic Aging Conditions
- The natural progression of the skin as we age
- The natural reduction of collagen, elastin, hyaluronic acid, proteins, etc.
- Dehydration due to loss of H20 production
- Loss of oil production, hence, no lubrication
- Sluggishness, slowing metabolism
- Sallow in color
- Pigmentation problems
- Genetics plays a big role in how we age intrinsically

Influenced Aging Factors
- Sun exposure
- Lack of proper care
- Poor diet and exercise
- Alcohol/Drug consumption
- Smoking
- Illness
- Medications
- Use of improper topicals

The Signs of Premature Aging

Most consider accumulated exposure to the sun as being the primary cause of premature aging, typically indicated by rough, leathery skin with fine wrinkles, loose skin, blotchy complexion, vascular damage, and uneven color/ dark spots. Other external contributing factors to premature aging include smoking, dehydration, and lack of sleep, all of which induce changes that affect the body's ability to eliminate oxidative damage and promote cellular repair.

Structural changes occur with inflammation and premature aging of the skin. Inflammation stimulates the production of free radicals, and once they are prevalent, the skin can no longer keep up with destroying them, resulting in cellular degradation. The abundance of free radicals inhibits elastin and collagen production, blocks the breakdown of melanocytes, which produce pigment, and diminish tissue repair and cellular proliferation.

Visible skin aging can be minimized and prevented by the daily use of anti-inflammatory products, coupled with an anti-inflammatory rich diet. The idea of avoiding and reversing chronic inflammation for the prevention and treatment of aging cells also applies to the skin's surface. It follows that skin cells would be expected to benefit from direct exposure to anti-inflammatory and antioxidant-containing topical skin care products, oral supplements and foods. To make significant improvements in the tone and texture of aging skin, you need to soothe inflammation on two fronts:

- By neutralizing free radicals (both inside and out)
- By boosting immune function through good nutrition, supplements, hormonal balance, detoxification, and topical support

How is Premature Aging Skin Treated?

The effects of premature aging can start with a myriad of factors that can happen over the course of time – and these conditions cannot be expected to improve with a single treatment. Multiple treatments are needed to achieve lasting results. A more effective multidimensional approach includes treatment, maintenance, and future prevention. The three goals when treating prematurely aging skin are as follows:

1. Exfoliate
The damaged epidermal layer can be gently removed through exfoliation, as well as increase cellular turnover, resulting in a fresher, healthier appearance.

2. Nourish
Prescribe products that provide solutions to treat inflammation and manage photo damage and oxidative stress. Hydrate and replenish the skin with topical products.

3. Protect
Sunblock protection in any routine is critical to successful treatment.

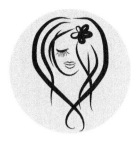

Understanding Acne & Its Treatment

Just the Facts...

- *Did you know that acne is affecting more than 60 million people in the United States?*
- *Over 80% of the population is affected during their teen years.*
- *Almost everyone will have acne, most get mild cases, some moderate and a few are severe.*

How Do I Handle Acne Clients?

With literally hundreds of different acne treatments available to choose from, it can be very confusing trying to decide what works and what doesn't. My mission today is to provide you with information to help you deal with your acne-prone clients. There are many different ways to not only treat acne, but also to prevent it before it occurs.

Acne should be approached as a chronic disease, which requires active treatment and a maintenance program to best stay in control of the condition.

How Does Acne Occur?

Many factors play a role in the connection of acne, including:
- A hereditary predisposition
- Effect of hormones
- After puberty, hormones stimulate the sebaceous glands to increase their size and produce more sebum
- The sebum is a good breeding ground for certain bacteria, which in turn produces inflammation within the hair follicle and the surrounding skin

• Depending upon the severity of the inflammation, the types of acne also vary in different individuals and at different times in the same individual

What is the Age Occurrence of Acne?

Contrary to popular belief, acne can occur at any age, from neonates to old age. Mostly acne is seen in early puberty to early adulthood, i.e., the ages of 12 to 25 years. About 50% of teenage acne can continue to adulthood. Some people, especially females, tend to have occasional flare-ups into their 30s. At the age of 40, 1% of males and 5% of females still have active lesions of acne.

Whiteheads and blackheads are the earliest skin lesions in acne. Depending upon the severity, acne is divided into **4 different types of acne:**

1. Comedonal
2. Papular
3. Pustular
4. Nodulocystic

Early treatment of acne may prevent scarring and it is important to select appropriate therapies according to the client's stage of the acne. Although the precise mechanisms of acne are not known, it is clearly accepted that there are these **four major factors involved in development of acne:**

1. An increased sebum production.
2. Hyperproliferation of ductal epidermis. Hypercornification is overproduction of epithelial cells lining follicles (sebaceous ducts, these ducts conduct sebum to the skin). Hypercornification may result in closure of the ducts and cause comedone and acne.
3. Bacterial colonization of the duct with Propionbacterium bacteria.
4. Further production of inflammation in acne sites.

Where does Acne Occur? How Does it Manifest?

Clients almost always exhibit acne on the face. Smaller percentages display acne on the back and on the chest. **Acne lesions are divided in two major groups.** Non-inflammatory and Inflammatory occurrences.
Treatment of these two types of acne may vary.

1. **Non-inflammatory lesions** or comedones are subdivided into whiteheads and blackheads.
   – Whiteheads are closed comedones with some accumulation of keratinized cell growth over the follicle, which results in closure of the follicle.
   – Blackheads or open comedones present as an obvious black lesion especially on the top. These are typically 1-3 mm in diameter.
   – Accumulation of the melanin (skin pigment) in blackheads cause the black color.

2. **Inflammatory lesions** such as papules, pustules, nodules, or cysts are among other manifestations of acne. Papules and pustules are more superficial compare to the rest of inflammatory acne, and their improvement takes a shorter period of time, 5-10 days. These pimples are caused by blockage of oil glands.
   – Papules are red lesions (pimples) that are similar to pustules but with a central collection of white pus at their top.

   Cysts are not very common but when they occur, they may reach several centimeters in diameter. Cysts are tender, sensitive, deeper and larger pimples filled with pus. Cystic acne is considered a severe acne form and its treatment must be consulted with a physician. Cystic acne improvement may take a longer period of time, and its recurrence is very likely.

Myths & Misconceptions of Acne

Though acne is the most common skin disease affecting more than 85% of the world's population at least once in their lifetime, there are many misconceptions and myths.

Foods and Acne

It has been known that certain food items like milk and milk products, sweets and oily food, could induce acne outbreaks and play a role in maintaining the acne condition. Many clinical studies and articles point toward the definite role of food in the beginning, progress and fuel of acne, at least in a portion of the sufferers.

Can Acne be Cured?

That acne can be cured is a definite myth. There is no cure for acne; it can only be controlled with prolonged treatment, maintenance services and topical home acne products.

Can Acne be Considered a Chronic Disease?

Acne starts around puberty and can run a continued course, even into the client's thirties. Acne can cause serious psychological and social impact in the affected. Delayed or improper treatment of acne can result in unwanted conditions, like scarring, post inflammatory pigmentation, and tissue disfiguration of the skin.

What other Skin Conditions can Mimic Acne?

- **Rosacea**
  – This condition can be characterized by acne-appearing pustules but not comedones, and occurs in the middle third of the face, along with redness, flushing, and superficial blood vessels. It generally affects people in their 30s and 40s and older.

- **Pseudofolliculitis** *sometimes called "razor bumps" or "razor rash"*
  – When cut close to the skin, curly neck hairs bend under the skin and produce small pimple-like bumps.

- **Folliculitis**
  – Pimples can occur on other parts of the body, such as the abdomen, buttocks, or legs. These represent not acne, but inflamed follicles.

How is Acne Skin Treated?

There is no single best mode for treatment of all lesions. Different treatments for different forms of acne is determined by many factors, including:
  – The type of lesions present
  – Duration of the acne
  – Past and present response(s) to treatment
  – Tendency for post-inflammatory hyper-pigmentation (PIH)

Knowing the symptoms and treating acne early and adequately are the keys to a successful acne management. Current medical condition and medications especially oral contraceptives, corticosteroids and topical antibiotics may affect its treatment. The client's overall current hygiene habits, facial care, use of cosmetics, and lifestyle must be considered.

There are two important points that acne patients should be aware of:
I always start by educating my acne clients that six to eight weeks of treatment may be required before improvement is noted. Also, remember that body lesions including back, chest, and shoulder areas respond more slowly to services and topical applications, than do those on the face.

My Approach to Treating Acne

First and foremost, I educate the client on the prevention of skin congestion/comedones. This tends to be the genesis for most acne conditions. Keeping their skin clean and well exfoliated is key. I like to get them started with a few "conditioning" or "detoxifying" facials, focusing on extractions to really clean the pores out. The home care regimen should start with two key products: Salicylic Acid (which creates an antimicrobial environment, dislodges the debris from the pores, and acts as an excellent anti-inflammatory agent) and Hyaluronic Acid (it is important to keep the skin well hydrated so that it can respond better to topicals and function at its optimum).

Second, it is important to control/reduce their oil (sebum) production. This can be accomplished with a home care regimen that contains Salicylic Acid. Balancing out the flow of oil can also be done with daily use of Hyaluronic Acid.

Third, preventing rupture of comedones. Making sure that they stay on top of the comedone and congestion with regular facials and products at home to eliminate the potential for bacterial inflammation, which can lead to scarring.

Fourth, keeping the red out! Keep inflammation low with anti-inflammatory topicals at home.

Fifth, preventing acne scars. It is easier to prevent than to correct the aftermath of acne. Keeping the skin clean, exfoliated, hydrated, and non-inflamed is the key!

Acne Service/Treatment Options

I successfully use the following modalities in the treatment of mild to severe acne, depending on the client, their conditions, budget, etc. These professional services are suggested to be used in conjunction with the appropriate home care regimen for best results.

- **Detoxifying Facials with Comedone Extractions** – Keep the pores clean!

- **Light Chemical Peels** – Improves acne by removing dead skin cells and helping to clear pores of debris. Estheticians may incorporate chemical peels into a facial for those with mild to moderate acne.

- **Microdermabrasion** – This treatment deeply exfoliates the skin, loosening debris from within the pore. It is best for those who have non-inflamed acne, whereas an inflamed acne condition could be aggravated and also can be uncomfortable for the inflamed acne clients.

- **Phototherapy** *(utilizing laser or light)* – Kills P. acnes bacteria, reducing inflammation, or shrinking the sebaceous glands, depending on what therapy is used. There are many different light and laser treatments available including blue light, red light, and photodynamic therapy. Phototherapy can be used to treat all stages of acne, from mild to very severe.

Example of Acne Program

This program is the combination of a series of acne facials and peels along with a home care regimen designed to correct acneic conditions.

 I strongly recommend at least **2 Detoxifying Facials**, a month apart.

 If the client is a good candidate for peels, for the third visit I add a **Salicylic Acid Peel** to my facial regimen.

 Once I realize that they can handle the peel ok, depending on the sensitivity levels and conditions present at the time, I then strongly recommend the **Fast-Track Peel Series**.

 Stand-alone Salicylic Acid Peels once every 2 weeks for 6 consecutive visits.

 Lastly, **Once-a-Month Facial with a Peel** added, for maintenance.

The Key Topical Acne Anecdotes for Home Care

Salicylic Acid's ability to slow down sebum activity justifies its value in acne. It also has an amazing keratolytic activity, causing peeling and removal of top layer of the skin and cell proliferation. This prevents the follicles from getting plugged. Salicylic Acid is also moderately effective in destroying Propionibacterium acnes and shows moderate antibacterial efficacy.

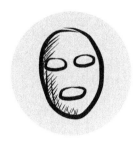

Understanding Pigmentation & Its Treatment

There are two categories of pigmentation disorders in the skin:

- Hypo-Pigmentation – The lack of pigment in the skin
- Hyper-Pigmentation – An overabundance of pigmentation in the skin

Hypo–Pigmentation

Hypo-Pigmentation is impossible for us, as Estheticians, to treat as it normally takes topical prescribed medications when and if it is possible to achieve results. Hyper-pigmentation CAN be successfully improved in variable degrees in most cases by some topical products and skin treatments. Here are the different types of hypo-pigmentation (decrease in skin pigmentation).

- **Pityriasis Alba** – Hypo-pigmented patch may be seen on the face usually in young children. It is common in winter and it can be treated with a mild topical steroid prescribed by a physician.

- **Pityriasis Versicolor** – It is a superficial fungal infection caused by a yeast. A well-defined hypo or hyper-pigmented lesions with fine scales are found on the chest, back, neck and sometimes on the face. It is treated with topical and oral antifungal drugs prescribed by a physician.

- **Leprosy** – It is a chronic disease caused by 'mycobacterium leprae' and affects mainly the skin and nerves. It can be cured with the help of drugs prescribed by a physician.

- **Vitiligo** – This is an autoimmune disease where de-pigmented patches are seen; they may occur anywhere on the body.

- **Post Inflammatory Hypo-Pigmentation** – It occurs after the healing phase of certain dermatoses such as eczemas, psoriasis, candidiasis, etc.

Hyper–Pigmentation

Hyper-Pigmentation may be due either to increased melanin deposition in the epidermis or dermis. These pigmentation types are usually close to the surface of the skin and are induced by sun exposure. Dermal (deep) pigmentation types are usually found in the dermal layers and are typically caused by trauma, injury, or lesions. Mixed dermal/epidermal pigmentation traverse through both the superficial and deeper layers of the skin. Epidermal pigmentary disorders respond well to treatment, while dermal pigmentation may take a long time to lighten.

Types of Hyper-Pigmentation Lesions:

- **Melasma** – Seen as brown patches on the face, it is more commonly seen in females. It occurs due to hormonal changes in the body. The pigmentation increases with sun exposure. *(Epidermis & Dermis)*

- **Peri-Orbital Melanosis** – Also known as 'dark circles' may be heriditary, due to stress, or eye strain. *(Can be found in both Epidermis & Dermis)*

- **Freckles and Lentigenes** – These are tiny black spots on the face and are genetic in origin. *(Dermis)*

- **Photomelanosis** – This is increased pigmentation due to sun exposure. The pigmentation occurs on exposed skin, commonly on the face, neck and back. The pigmentation may be patchy or diffused darkening of the exposed skin. *(Can be both Epidermis & Dermis)*

- **Sunburn (tan)** – A condition commonly encountered in fair skinned people due to excessive sun exposure. *(Can be both Epidermis & Dermis, depending on severity of burn)*

- **Post Inflammatory Hyper-Pigmentation** – It may be seen in the following cases. *(Can be both Epidermis & Dermis)*
  - Seen after healing has occurred, like in acne, eczemas, contact dermatitis, etc.
  - Drug induced pigmentation.
  - Pigmentation due to cosmetics especially those containing fragrance.

- **Nevus or 'Birth Mark'** – Usually seen at birth, but may also appear at a later age.

How is Pigmentation Treated?

How do treatments and products work to lighten pigmentation? The first method of treating skin pigmentation is to prevent its appearance or worsening existing pigmentation by diligent, daily use of sun protection. UV exposure from sunlight or sun beds will invariably worsen any existing pigmentation, and promote further pigmentation to arise. Furthermore, sunscreen should be applied every day, even if it is cloudy or overcast, as UV light is still present. It is also important to avoid direct sunlight, especially during the middle hours of the day, seek shade when possible, and wear a hat and protective clothing.

Topical lightening agents can be used in conjunction to help reduce skin pigmentation. Topical lightening agents help to reduce pigmentation by inhibiting enzymes that produce melanin (skin pigment), and by increasing the turnover of the skin to flush out existing pigmentation.

What skin lighteners are safe? The marketplace is full of skin lightening products that contain dangerous and potentially harmful chemicals like Hydroquinone and Mercury. Products containing these ingredients have been banned in some countries because of potential health risks. I strongly suggest avoiding these ingredients. The safest alternative ingredient is Alpha Arbutin, derived from bearberry extract.

What is the treatment for Hyper-Pigmented disorders?

For best results, we must treat hyper-pigmentation two-fold; in treatment and home care.

For Professional Treatments I recommend:
A **Glycolic Acid** and/or **Lactic Acid** peel program (depending on the sensitivity levels of the skin, 6 or more treatments at two-week intervals)

For Home Care I recommend:
Lactic Acid, Alpha Arbutin and **Sun Protection**

Rosacea...The Silent Aging Condition

During my research, I was shocked to discover that an estimated 16 million Americans have rosacea! Six out of ten clients that we see have some type of rosacea, from mild to severe. Rosacea is a chronic and potentially life-disruptive disorder primarily of the facial skin. Many have observed that it typically begins any time after age 30 as redness on the cheeks, nose, chin or forehead, and may come and go. In some cases, rosacea may also occur on the neck, chest, scalp or ears. Over time, the redness tends to become ruddier and more persistent, and visible blood vessels may appear. If left untreated, bumps and pimples often develop, and in severe cases the nose may grow swollen and bumpy from excess tissue.

Various theories about the disorder's origin have evolved over the years. We do know that when present, this disorder causes facial blood vessels to dilate easily, and the increased blood near the skin surface makes the skin appear red and flushed. Various things I called "stingers" can increase this response such as heat, some products, foods, etc. Acne-like bumps can appear, often in the center of the face. Some specialists believe that the following should be considered as potential causes: poor blood flow, bacteria, irritation of follicles, sun damage of the connective tissue, an abnormal immune or inflammatory response, or psychological factors.

Although rosacea can affect us across all segments of the population, individuals with fair skin who tend to flush or blush easily are believed to be at greatest risk. The disease is more frequently diagnosed in women, but more severe symptoms tend to be seen in men. While there is currently no cure for rosacea and the cause is somewhat unknown, topical and oral medications are available to control or reverse its signs and symptoms. Individuals who suspect they may have rosacea are urged to see a dermatologist or other knowledgeable physician for diagnosis and appropriate treatment.

Rosacea can vary substantially from one individual to another, and in most cases, always includes at least one of the following signs and/or symptoms. Persistent facial redness is the most common individual sign of rosacea, and may resemble a blush or sunburn that does not go away.

- Small red solid bumps or pimples often develop. Burning or stinging may occur.
- With many rosacea sufferers, small blood vessels become visible on the skin.
- Burning or stinging sensations may often occur on the face. Itching or a feeling of tightness may also develop.
- The central facial skin may be rough and very dry.
- Raised red patches, known as plaques, may develop without changes in the surrounding skin.
- The skin may thicken and enlarge from excess tissue, most commonly on the nose. This condition, known as rhinophyma, affects more men than women.
- Facial swelling may accompany other signs of rosacea, or occur independently.

Although no scientific research has been performed on rosacea and heredity, there is evidence that suggests rosacea may be inherited. Nearly 40 percent of rosacea patients surveyed by the National Rosacea Society said they could name a relative who had similar symptoms. In addition, what I thought was interesting is that there are strong signs that ethnicity may also be a factor. In a separate survey by the Rosacea Society, 33 percent of respondents reported having at least one parent of Irish heritage, and 26 percent had a parent of English descent. Other ethnic groups with elevated rates of rosacea compared with the U.S. population as whole, included individuals of Scandinavian, Scottish, Welsh or Eastern European descent.

Rosacea is a chronic disorder, rather than a short-term condition, and is often characterized by relapses and remissions. While at present there is no cure for rosacea, its symptoms can usually be controlled with medical therapy and lifestyle modifications. Moreover, studies have shown that rosacea patients who continue therapy for the long-term are less likely to experience a recurrence of symptoms.

We have to remember that within our scope of practice we cannot diagnose any skin diseases or disorders. It is best to collaborate with a local Dermatologist on ways that we can help to relieve or improve the symptoms associated with the skin disorder.

Because the signs and symptoms of rosacea vary from one patient to another, treatment must be tailored by a physician for each individual case. Various oral and topical medications may be prescribed to treat the bumps, pimples and redness often associated with the disorder. Dermatologists often prescribe initial treatment with oral and topical therapy to bring the condition under immediate control, followed by long-term use of the topical therapy alone to maintain remission.

In addition to medical therapy, rosacea patients can improve their chances of maintaining remission by identifying and avoiding lifestyle and environmental factors that may trigger flare-ups or aggravate their individual conditions. Identifying these factors is an individual process, however, because what causes a flare-up for one person may have no effect on another.

Proper Skin Care & Cosmetics

- Consistent, gentle skin care and effective use of makeup can make a visible difference in managing rosacea and improving the look of your client's skin.
- The key is to use products and techniques that minimize irritation. One good guide – look for products that are noted as appropriate for sensitive skin or skin with rosacea - and avoid any products that sting, burn or cause irritation.
- In a National Rosacea Society survey of 1,066 patients, 41 percent reported that certain skin care products aggravated their condition and 27 percent said certain cosmetics also caused rosacea flare-ups.

To avoid irritation, follow these tips when choosing skin care and makeup products:

Watch out for common rosacea irritants. In surveys conducted by the National Rosacea Society, many patients cited the following ingredients as triggers for irritation:

- Alcohol (66%)
- Witch Hazel (30%)
- Fragrance (30%)
- Menthol (21%)
- Peppermint (14%)
- Eucalyptus Oil (13%)

Most Rosacea sufferers said they avoided astringents, exfoliating agents and other types of products that may be too harsh for sensitive skin.

- Choose fragrance-free skin care and makeup products. According to the American Academy of Dermatology, "Fragrances cause more allergic contact dermatitis than any other ingredient." Skin is a vast portal for allergens, and the irritations allergies bring can weaken skin even more. Using fragrance-free and allergy-tested products reduces your risk of skin irritation. Note that "allergy tested" shouldn't be confused with "hypoallergenic", a term that is not clearly defined by the cosmetics industry.

- Test a product first. Before using a product on your face, try it on a patch of skin in a peripheral area, such as the neck. If you have a reaction, avoid the product and note the ingredients. Rosacea irritants may vary from person to person, so your individual skin's reaction should be your guide.

- Use minimal products. Rosacea patients should also consider reducing the number of items they use on their skin by choosing products with multiple functions.

FROM BEHIND THE CHAIR...
TIPS OF THE TRADE

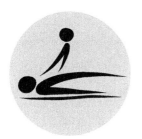

Extraction Tips & Techniques

Most facials are relaxing, luxuriant and painless. They involve steam, exfoliating and gentle massage, and most skin care practitioners can perform them well.

Clinical facials, however, are a slightly different story. They can be uncomfortable, and they require a higher level of expertise. The difference is the extractions and the tools that you use.

Extractions are a necessary step within the facial for the purpose of drawing out pore-clogging sebum, using a precise technique and gentle pressure – without scarring or tearing the skin. With luck, the plug of sebaceous matter is coaxed from the pore. Not only do extractions immediately improve the look of the skin (especially if the blackhead was large and obvious), but done regularly, they can help reduce breakouts.

To Extract or Not to Extract
- First of all, your state regulations need to be reviewed. Some states allow tools, when others don't, some allow lancets and others don't.
- ALWAYS PROTECT YOURSELF with gloves and masks if necessary.

Why Extractions?
- The goal is to leave the skin looking and feeling clean, clear, and healthy. Facials that don't include extractions will not accomplish this goal.
- If the filament remains inside the pores, bacteria festers and acne lesions could occur.
- Also, the pore openings can be permanently stretched by the clogging matter.
- As the comedones are full of acids, bacteria and other material, such as dead skin cells, scarring could be the end result if left untreated.

- There's no doubt that extractions can be a major ally in the quest for smooth, clear skin.
- Getting that sebum out of the pore can flatten the bump, reduce the irritation, and make pores appear smaller.

There are 4 Types of Lesions that We can Extract

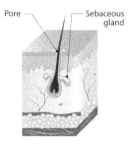

Closed Comedone – A plug that stays under the skin and appears as a little white bump (commonly called a whitehead).

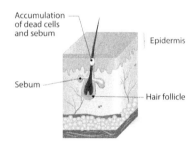

Open Comedone – A plug that reaches the skin surface and opens up. It may look like a black speck of dirt (and is commonly called a blackhead).

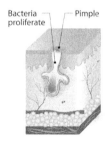

Papules – Small pink bumps on the skin surface that may be tender when touched (also called inflamed comedones).

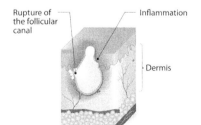

Pustules – Red skin bumps filled with yellow or white pus (commonly called pimples).

When Should We Extract?
- Only when a prominent open lesion is present do we perform extractions.
- Prepping the skin is mandatory in order to soften the filament for fewer traumas to the skin, and to liquefy the filament so it is easily extracted.

When Shouldn't We Extract?
- Cystic Acne is severe acne with the formation of cysts enclosing a mixture of keratin and sebum in varying proportions. Cystic acne is more likely to leave scars and should be treated by a Dermatologist. Cysts are beyond our license and scope of practice.

How Do We Extract Properly?
Extractions require some skill to do correctly. Finger or tool placement, appropriate pressure, and squeezing techniques need to be polished in order to successfully extract. There are two methods, but there are many various extraction techniques, and each individual may benefit from a different type.
- Manually
- Using a Tool

Properly Prepare! Have all of your supplies handy and ready to go.
You will need the following accessible on your cart:
- Gloves
- 4 x 4s
- Extraction Tool (if desired)
- Q-Tips
- Extraction Prep Solution
- Post Extraction Anti-Microbial

Preparing the Skin Prior to Extractions
The skin must be properly prepared before beginning extractions.
- Soften the debris in the pores as much as possible prior to extractions with stream and/or warm towels to avoid trauma on the skin.
- Protect the client's eyes from the mag light with eye pads.
- Apply some type of enzyme, keratolytic or exfoliant for 7-10 minutes with steam to soften the filament.
- Apply the softening agent to the area that you are extracting. Leave on for 1 minute.
- Keep the skin moist throughout the extractions.

Performing the Extractions
I have designed what I call the **4 Methods of Extraction**. The method that you choose can be determined by preference, however, I find that it is more relevant to the type and stage of the acne lesion that persuades me to make the choice of what technique is best.

My Different Methods of Manual Extractions:

The "Squeeze" Technique
This method simply comes at the comedone or plug horizontally and simultaneously from each side applying light pressure. This method is for those "ready to be extracted" lesions as it's a mild, gentle approach. Be sure that there is a follicular opening whereas the filament and fluid can easily evacuate from the pore without tearing the growth of skin that may be covering the pore opening. If not, this could result in tissue scarring. I prefer this method for a more grade 3 acne, where inflammation or pustular activity is present.

The *"Wiggle"* Technique

This method is best used when comedones or pore filament need to be "coaxed" out of the pore. This method is helpful for the removal of deeply lodged, old, dry comedones by simply placing both index fingers to each side of the comedone and create a back and forth movement.

Note: Keeping the skin moist for this method can really help! Spritz the skin with hydrator throughout the process of loosening the debris from the pore.

The *"Scooping"* Technique

This method is ideal when there is an obvious, large comedone or plug, whereas you can actually get under the "nodule" with your fingers and squeeze up and out with a bit more pressure. I usually only use this method when there isn't any discomfort or inflammation present.

The *"Scaling"* Technique

One of my favorite techniques. This is best used with a pre-extraction product to soften the filament and debris first. Keep the skin moist throughout this method. Using the long side or edge of your comedone extractor, slide the tool gently but with a bit of pressure across the surface of the skin to remove the congestion. I love this method on larger areas that have many small, white plugs in the skin, or on contoured areas like the nose.

Extractions Gone Bad

When this acne treatment is done correctly – by a professional in a sterile environment – it's a safe procedure. Acne extraction can quickly clear up unsightly acne, and over time, even help prevent future acne breakouts when other preventive measures, like proper skin cleaning and correctors are also used. Also, if acne extraction is not professionally handled, there are some serious risks involved. Extracting incorrectly, such as with pressure that's too firm or in the wrong direction, can lead to:

— A bacterial infection of the skin
— Increased irritation
— Vascular damage
— In a worst-case scenario, inappropriate extractions can even cause infection and scarring

Poorly performed extractions can also be pretty painful. When done correctly, extractions may be a little uncomfortable, but shouldn't hurt.

How much should I extract per visit? Create a plan. You must decide how many treatments it will take to successfully extract what needs to be extracted. Discuss with your client. Request multiple treatments if necessary.

- Try not to extract for more than 15 minutes per facial. If more time is necessary, you may cut back on massage time. In some cases, with inflamed acne, massage may be eliminated all together so that you can focus on the extraction process more.

Follow Up Care

- While extracting, follow each extraction with a dab of an antibacterial agent with a disposable, cotton tip applicator. This will disinfect the area, tighten up the appearance of the pore, and reduce inflammation.
- Be sure to finish the treatment off with a cooling, soothing, anti-inflammatory mask.

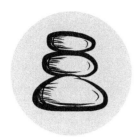

Mastering the Magic of Facial Massage

Mastering the art of your facial massage is a critical piece to most esthetic treatments. Throughout my years of teaching, I have always been asked to provide the protocol that I perform. So, here it is!

- Turn your steamer on at least 3 minutes prior to massage.
- Pump 2 pumps of your massage oil into the palms of your hands. Warm up oil under the steam.
- Apply a layer of the oil everywhere you will be working (sternum, deltoids, upper traps, neck, chin, cheeks, forehead).
- You will always be working in upward strokes, each stroke is designed to flow one into the next with continuous movement.

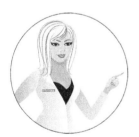

LESSON #20

"Mastering the art of your facial massage is a critical piece to most esthetic treatments."

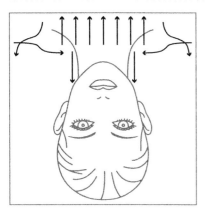

Stroke #1

Massage along the lower edge of the clavicle, massage down around the deltoids and onto the back of the neck. Repeat 5-8 times. Without losing contact, go right into stroke #2.

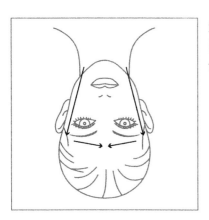

Stroke #2

Begin by sliding up the sides of the face simultaneously, and onto the center of the forehead.

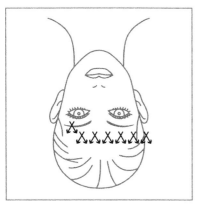

Stroke #3

Begin to crisscross to the left and back to the right. Repeat 4 times. End up in the center.

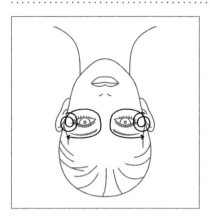

Stroke #4

Using circular strokes, do circular motions on the outside of the right eye three times, and then around the entire eye. Repeat 4 times. Then switch to the left eye and repeat without losing contact.

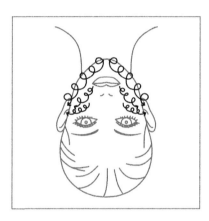

Stroke #5

Slide down to the jaw bone and using circular motions, starting at the center of the chin, use simultaneous upward circles on each side to the ears, then slide to the corners of the mouth and using circular motions outward to the ears, and then to the sides of the nose, use circular motions outward to the ears and back down to chin. Repeat 4 times.

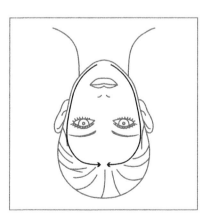

Stroke #6

Using longer strokes, begin at the chin by scissoring middle and forefingers on the jaw bone and alternate side to side. Repeat 6 times on each side.

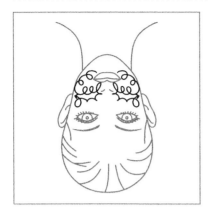

Stroke #7

Using middle finger, use circular motions on the cheeks with fingertips and/or knuckles and on the side of the cheeks working up and down and all around the cheek and front of the face in small circles. Massage the earlobe in between the middle and thumb.

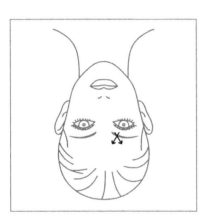

Stroke #8

Criss-cross thumbs at the eyebrows above the nose.

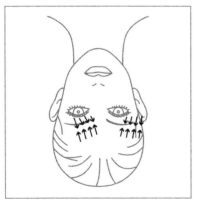

Stroke #9

Eyebrow pinch – take tissue of eyebrows and pinch tissue between index finger and thumb, working medially to laterally, ending at temple.

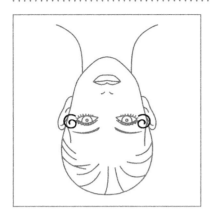

Stroke #10

Temple circles.

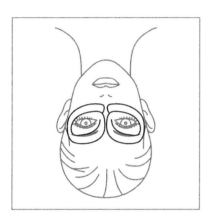

Stroke #11

Eye orbits – with fingertips leaving the temples, go around forehead and circle around eyes, being careful not to pull delicate eye tissue. Repeat 3-5 times.

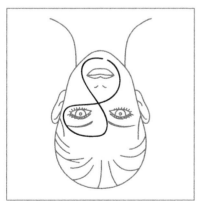

Stroke #12

Hourglass stroke – begin at the medial aspect of the base of the chin. Stroke upward in the shape of an hourglass to just below the zygomatic arch, back out and up to the forehead. Repeat 3-5 times.

SALES &
MAR-
KET-
ING

Becoming a Retail Specialist

Retailing is absolutely a lifeline to success in this industry. How do you maximize your earning potential? By selling retail products! Remember these 3 things…

- Plant the seed…develop the need. Suggestive selling works! Tell your clients what they need and why.
- Make it attractive…how do they benefit from what it is you're selling?
- Assume the sale! You've got this! Teach them what you know!

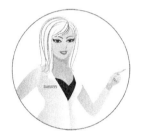

LESSON #21

"Our clients should always feel served, not sold."

The Art of Selling Through Education

Selling products can double, if not triple, your revenues and commissions. Remember, in a spa we can cap out per hour per room if we think one-dimensional. Selling multiple products with very little added time or effort is one of the two only *real* growth potential efforts in the long run.

There are **6 major concerns** that you are likely to encounter when retailing. The client has:

- No Need for Your Products/Services
- No Trust in You
- No Interest in Your Products/Services
- No Hurry to Buy
- No Ability to Decide
- No Ability to Pay

When selling, you must think about and identify which concern(s) they have. Create solutions for their concerns and give them enough education to make a buying decision. We have several opportunities to educate/sell to our clients.

Before the Service

The consultation time is the simplest way to retail. Ask the following important questions, as their answers will spell out exactly what they are looking for and what their expectations are:

- What would they like to see improved with their skin?
- What do they like about the products they use?
- What don't they like?

Be sure to identify the difference between urgent and important. Do they need it to get the results they want? Next, suggestive sell the recommended home care regimen and treatment plan that you have formulated to achieve their goals.

Throughout the Service

I practice what I call "permission-based selling". That just means that I ask before I assume they want to learn from me. Most will say yes. At that time, always describe what you are doing and with what. Describe the benefits of each step and product of the service. Gently describe how they can extend the results of the service at home with a quality skin care regimen customized for them.

ALWAYS Have Your Clients Bring in the Products That They Currently Use!

This way we can tell so much more about our clients:

- See what they buy
- How much they spend
- Why they buy
- Are they a minimalist or a junkie?
- Determine their immediate needs

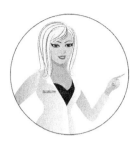

LESSON #22
"Great selling is a byproduct of great service."

Here are some of the sales killers that I have experienced. When we...
- Fail to build a rapport with our client.
- Fail to determine our client's needs.
- Focus on our own agenda instead of the client's needs.
- Don't give our client the majority of the talking time.
- Confuse "telling" with "selling".
- Don't listen or hear what client is saying.
- Don't know our promotions, specials and regular pricing.
- Don't differentiate our product/service enough to create value in the mind of the client.
- Sell too fast, trying to close a sale before the client is ready to buy.
- Fail to address our client's objections properly, not realizing that providing a resolution to our client's concern(s) is the quickest way to get them to purchase.

Think about **selling benefits not products.** What it does, not what it is! Clients always want to know what's in it for them! They are less inclined to make a buying decision because of the technical part of the product or service, but become more enthusiastic about a product or service if they think they can benefit somehow from it.

Show your passion when you describe your products! Provide your client with an **opportunity to make a buying decision.** I cannot stress enough the importance of product knowledge when it comes to making sales. Those who have learned everything they can about the products they sell have a distinct advantage over those who don't. Given the option, clients would choose to talk to the person who knows the most about the product they are considering. Good product knowledge will help even the most reserved Esthetician. Knowledge gives us confidence knowing that we have something of value to tell the client.

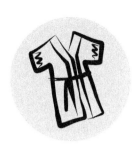

Marketing Yourself for Success
Ideas to Build Your Practice

First things first. If you are just starting out or looking to expand your current client list, we have to continue to **fill your pipeline with prospective clients.** Start with the people that you know. This group could be made up of several friends and family, neighbors, and people you do business with. You may want to offer a special limited-time discount to any of these people.

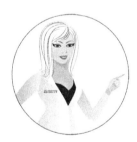

LESSON #23

"You, as an individual, are really the biggest marketing piece for your business; and your personality, ambition and tenacity will likely attract the type of clientele you attract."

Always network with people you meet! Networking is basically about meeting people and exchanging information with one another in the hopes of benefiting each other and each other's businesses. There are many groups in existence designed just for networking, but you can also network at work, social gatherings, even at the grocery store. The key is to always carry plenty of business cards and be prepared to talk about what you do.

Focus on referrals and word-of-mouth advertising. Referrals and word-of-mouth advertising are by far the most effective and inexpensive ways to build a clientele. To get started, ask your current clients and the people you know to send you prospects. You can also ask for referrals from other related professionals, such as a chiropractor, hair salon, yoga instructor, etc. Offer a special discount or incentive for each person they refer, and be sure to deliver that incentive promptly with a 'thank you'.

Conventional advertising isn't always the best form of advertising for our industry, other than to establish your branding in your very local market. The most powerful form of advertising in our market is word-of-mouth since it is a *personal, touch, feel service-based business.* Most potential clients will find us through referrals - by talking to their friends, family members or other service professionals, such as hairdressers or physicians.

If you choose to try to attract new clients with the traditional printed ad method, do your research and understand exactly what you are buying, and how it will potentially benefit your business. Be realistic about the returns and remember that repetition is the key.

I also love to do local press releases, articles, and presentations, and have found these to be incredibly successful. This sort of advertising is usually low cost or free. Newspapers and local television shows are always looking for someone to interview, or for an interesting beauty-based story to share with their readers. Exposure of your business and professionalism through the media and public appearances will do more for your credibility than you know. The ways in which you can build your practice is really limitless. Building a clientele is not a one-stop experience, but rather a career-long endeavor that takes work and persistence.

There are several internal and external promotional strategies that also work very well. Here are a few that have been beneficial for me:

- Cross-Selling with Staff Members
- Up-Selling More Services to Existing Clients
- Events/Open Houses to Educate Clients on New Services, Products, etc.
- Product of the Month Promotion (New Product, Seasonal, etc.)
- Service of the Month Promotion (Seasonal, Holidays)
- Direct Mail
- Email
- External Local Events & Trade Shows

An additional promotional idea to stimulate product sales that works well is a product recycling/trade-in program with your clientele. Whether you do this as a one-time or ongoing program, offering a $5 or 10% discount for every product they replace with one of your products, has several benefits.

- First, you motivate clients to get rid of product that they probably don't use, and feel guilty about "just throwing it out".
- Second, you know that when they buy your products, they don't have a backup product to use in place of repurchasing your product.
- Third, you know they aren't going to interfere with your recommended home care regimen by inserting a product that contraindicates their condition.

Hosting private VIP events can be great to honor and recognize your best clients and reward them for their loyalty, and ensures the long-term relationship. Be sure to capture their testimonials at the event, in exchange for a free product or service.

Hosting or speaking at events is a sure way to build your book of business. Simply search a 5 mile radius from your spa on the internet for "Women's/ Men's Organizations". Write them a letter, call, or email them an introductory form letter introducing yourself, your business, your services and products. Let them know you are interested in speaking to their group about topics that spark interests, such as:

  – "How to Protect Your Skin From Premature Aging"
  – "Learn the Importance of Caring for Your Skin"
  – "How to Tackle Menopausal Acne/Breakouts"

Be sure to always present yourself through **EDUCATION**. Once they validate you as a credible, knowledgeable source, they will do business with you. Let them know that you can appear at their events, or you can possibly "host" their event at your spa. They all love to have guest speakers and places to hold their meetings!

In addition, **community networking** or what I call "tables in the community", is a great way to meet prospective clients face to face. Set up a table at a gym, organic food market, yoga/dance studios, trade shows, etc. Barter complimentary services to owners of these businesses to allow you to set up a table. Provide incentives for each passerby to stop and listen to what you are offering. Some form of audio/visual can be very powerful in these focused settings. Videos, demos, and some interaction is good.

Lastly, **become the local press darling for your industry!** Search the internet for media contacts in your demographic. Build a database of important contacts across all media sources; i.e. radio, television, newspaper, local city websites and guides, etc. Host a media event and invite them to attend. The goal is to inform them of a hot new product or service you are offering (tie it in with your monthly promotion), get them to write a column, article, blog, etc. about your business, or be picked up by the local television broadcasts. Write a press release and send it along with your cover letter with pictures/ images so they can do their research on your business and learn more about your business prior to attending, and to spark them to write about you. Take pictures at these events! Can be used on websites, social media sites, newsletters, portfolio books, etc.

Don't overlook the power of **Social Media!** You can take your business and brand to the next level by interacting with your clients where they already spend some of their time (Facebook, Instagram, Twitter and Pinterest – Google+ will help your Google search results). Create a look and personality on your pages – be recognizable. Be consistent with your brand name and message. You may also want to look into how to create a free webpage, including a Blog where you can share your expertise, and grow a following.

What to post?
- Skin Care Tips
- Anti-Aging Tips
- Inspirational Tips
- Ingredient Benefits

Don't forget to #Hashtag
#YourBusiness/BrandName
#SkinCareExpert
#BeautyExpert
#UniqueHashtag
#QOTD (quote of the day)

Have FUN and be CONFIDENT in your passion and expertise!

LET'S CONNECT!

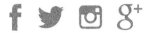

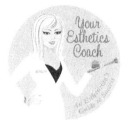

Facebook.com/YourEstheticsCoach
@YourEstheticsCoach
#YourEstheticsCoach
#KarlaKeene

Visit us at
YourEstheticsCoach.com

A one-stop site in which professional Estheticians like ourselves can gather and interact and empower each other, stay informed, receive quality, unbiased education and training, learn the latest technologies in our industry and more!

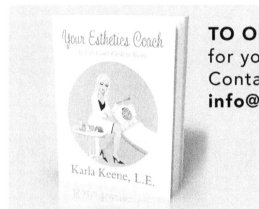

TO ORDER BOOKS
for your Group of 25 or more
Contact us at
info@yourestheticscoach.com

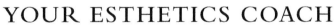

YOUR ESTHETICS COACH
A MENTOR & RESOURCE FOR MEDICAL ESTHETICS

To have Karla Keene Speak to your Group
Contact us at
info@yourestheticscoach.com

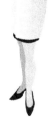

About Karla Keene, L.E.

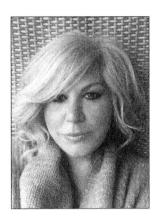

Karla Keene has volumes of practical experience working with cosmetic physicians, estheticians, clinicians, franchises, and entrepreneurs in this market, as well as with prominent product and equipment companies in a myriad of capacities. She has a proven track record with advanced education, profit-driven sales and account management success in the skin care, day spa, medspa and cosmetic medicine industry. She has served as part of several senior-level teams making decisions on strategic and tactical planning, product development, business development, national account development, brand management and new product and line extension launches for some of the industry's leading skin care companies for over 30 years. One of her career highlights is that she had the privilege of being the Lead Medical Esthetician for The Chief of Plastic Surgery at Cedar-Sinai in Beverly Hills, CA. very early in her career.

As a consultant to this industry, she has opened over 70 medical spas and has trained hundreds of clinicians, estheticians and spa/medspa owners. She also presently acts as an on-going consultant to one of the largest massage and facial spa franchises in the country where she created their original facial program, service menus, treatment protocols, and has had the pleasure of training over 2,500 estheticians, sales associates, and franchisees on clinical skin care, retail selling, business building, and the like to date. Karla has been a member of National Advisory Board for the Medical Spa Expo & Conferences as an education advisor responsible for ensuring quality advanced esthetic education. Karla is a published, best-selling author, and a frequent contributor to trade publications, industry resources and articles. She has been published/ quoted in prestigious national magazines, newspapers, and websites such as Wounds Magazine, New York Daily News, Allure Spa Magazine, Massage Magazine, MedEsthetics Magazine, Franchise News, and more. Karla is also still a practicing Licensed Cosmetologist/Esthetician at her ClarityRx Skin Wellness Boutique in Newport Beach, CA.

References

www.indeed.com; esthetician's statistics

http://en.wikipedia.org/wiki/Cosmetology#Esthetician; Scope of Practice

United States Food and Drug Administration (FDA), the Food, Drug, and Cosmetic Act

Dermatologist Dr. Leslie Baumann

Skin and the Effects of Aging – WebMD
www.webmd.com/beauty/aging/effects-of-aging-on-skin

American Academy of Dermatology

National Rosacea Society

Winter, Ruth M.S. (2005). A Consumer's Dictionary of Cosmetic Ingredients,

Three Rivers Press, NY. Cornell University: Parabens: evidence of estrogenicity and endocrine disruption Environmental Health Perspectives Volume 114, Number 12, December 2006

The US Environmental Protection Agency (EPA) report "Pharmaceuticals and Personal Care Products in the Environment: Agents of Subtle Change?"

Advanced Professional Skin Care Medical Edition Peter Pugliese, MD

This book is literally a compendium of knowledge, information, and informed experience-based insight acquired by the author over 30 years of multi-faceted involvement in the field. Every effort has been made to acknowledge the many experts and the many significant sources and resources that have helped to shape and inform this book, but a truly complete list is, for all practical purposes, impossible to assemble. The author is grateful for and indebted to them all.

Printed in Great Britain
by Amazon